FASTING

A PATH FOR HEALING, TRANSFORMATION & LIBERATION

ACHARYA SHREE YOGEESH

Siddha Sangh Publications

SIDDHA SANGH PUBLICATIONS
9985 E. HWY 56
Windom, Texas 75492
info@siddhayatan.org

Copyright © 2021 by Acharya Shree Yogeesh
Cover design: Sadhvi Anubhuti
Author photo: Alannah Avelin

www.siddhayatan.org
www.thefastingbook.com

ISBN - 978-17334750-2-0

Library of Congress Control Number - 2021915589

Disclaimer

Please note that not all exercises, diet plans, or other suggestions, mentioned in this book are suitable for everyone. This book is not intended to replace the need for consultation with medical doctors and other professionals. Before changing any diet, exercise routine, or any other plans discussed in this book, seek appropriate professional medical advice to ensure it is acceptable for you. The author and publisher are not responsible for any problems arising from the use or misuse of the information, materials, demonstrations or references provided in this book. Results are not guaranteed.

Printed in the United States of America.

TABLE OF CONTENTS

"Before meeting enlightened master Acharya Shree Yogeesh, I had no idea how important, precious, and powerful my body was...let alone my willpower. Through water fasting, I realized that I could go for more than 24 hours without food and survive quite well; I wouldn't say that it was a comfortable experience, but I will say that it was attainable and the end result was worth the temporary discomfort. Nonetheless, I realized that I had power over my sense of taste. Acharya Shree says that the biggest addiction is not drugs or alcohol, rather food, and I can personally vouch for that. I love snacking, especially on salty foods late in the evening. However, after breaking my water fast, I noticed that my cravings for unhealthy foods and unnecessary snacking ceased. I felt cleaner and lighter on the inside, and so I didn't want to put unhealthy food back into my system. By putting my willpower into practice through water fasting, I managed to increase it, as well as my self-confidence. Thanks to Acharya Shree's knowing, guidance, and support, I would have not discovered the power I held in my own hands this entire time. Having the ability to withstand hunger for such a long period of time not only shows how strong those who go hungry are but that we don't need as much as we are told we need. I believe that if you can abstain from food for at least 24 hours, you can accomplish anything! Acharya Shree is the greatest blessing in my life, and I am forever grateful to him!" — Riddhika N. | Regina, SK, Canada

"I met Acharya Shree Yogeesh in Estonia in 2014 and have been his student ever since. For me, his teachings were a qualitatively new approach to non-violence, human nature, and life in general. I got answers to many of my questions. Following his practical teachings has made me stronger, both physically and mentally, and has kept my body and mind healthy. If one is ready to follow his teachings, a lot of work needs to be done, especially within oneself. In order to make this world a little better place, Acharya Shree has taught me first to improve myself. This, in turn, requires an understanding of what needs to change first. Fasting is another special teaching of

Acharya Shree's. Before meeting the master, I fasted on herbal tea, water, and juice. But after meeting him, I tried dry fasting for the first time, and to my own surprise, it suited me best. I fast regularly once a month for one to two days and follow a vegetarian diet for years now. The more I detoxify my body, the easier fasting becomes. I have fewer challenges and can calmly continue with all the necessary daily activities. I also wanted to fast for a longer period of time, but it needed a suitable time and place. However, during the COVID-19 pandemic, I had time off from work, and because the pandemic required isolation, it became the perfect time to try it. I set a goal to fast for three weeks with the flexibility to interrupt it if necessary. I felt so good and achieved my goal. This time, I did not restrict my fast to water only. I had water, herbal teas, and during the third week, I had juices. Fasting is an intense opportunity to engage with oneself. It was important to move, practice Purnam Yoga, and do breathing exercises in the fresh air during my fast. It gave me a new charge for the day. Fasting has made my body lighter, not only by pounds but also by toxins, as well as making my mind clearer and burning karma. I know there is still a lot of work I must do with myself, but I know my efforts will fully pay off. My spiritual journey with self-discovery continues." — Amisha T. | Tallinn, Estonia

"Fasting is one of the most powerful spiritual practices that accelerates me to reconnect to my pure soul. Fasting ignites the willpower that resides within us. Fasting is like a fire that burns layers of layers of karma and uncovers the infinite creativities and wisdom within the self. I have infinite love and respect to Acharya Shree, my spiritual teacher, who taught me about fasting and guides me to the path of soul purification. I continue walking courageously to liberate my soul, as my soul has been calling to come back home: the home of oneness and total freedom. Jai Siddhatma!" — Kathy W. L. | Washington DC, USA

FOREWORD

In August of 2011, my life took a different turn after meeting and learning from my spiritual teacher and guru Acharya Shree Yogeesh. His universal teachings affected me profoundly. I remember when he told me that to change the world, I needed to change myself first. And that if I wanted to help others, I needed to help myself first. Often we desperately want to change the world or change others. But we never think about changing or helping ourselves. Instead of looking at others or on the outside, I needed to look at myself. Once I reversed the lens, I had a real look at what really needed to change. And that was *me*. But what about myself needed to change? Well, looking closely, I needed to change a lot of things. I needed to improve myself in many ways: my thinking, my attitude, my beliefs, my speech, my actions, my emotions, my health, my habits and so much more. There is an endless list of ways we can improve and there is also an endless list of ways we don't realize we need to improve.

During my first retreat at Siddhayatan Tirth & Spiritual Retreat, Acharya Shree taught me about *ahimsa*, or non-violence. I had never thought about the many ways we are violent day-to-day. Many of our traditions, beliefs, and habits can create violence and we are not aware of it. For example, I didn't know I was causing harm by the foods I was eating. It shook me to my core to realize that for 29 years of my life, many precious lives were taken to satisfy my palate. I was ignorant about it and wished I could go back in time to have learned about this much sooner. I could have avoided causing pain and death to the many animals served on my plate and avoided collecting karma during all those years. Thankfully, I understood the impact of eating animals right away, and since then, I promised myself that I would never eat them again.

The real concept of karma was another teaching Acharya Shree introduced me to. Karma was and continues to be one of the most fascinating things to learn about because it reveals many of life's mysteries and it answers my deepest questions. To be honest, I had no idea how much karma was blocking my soul. Every day we collect new karma, and if we are unaware of it, we just keep engulfing ourselves with more karma. I felt so much relief when I learned there are ways to stop it and eliminate it. But I knew it would take time and require a lot of work.

When Acharya Shree introduced me to the teachings of fasting, things didn't click for me right away. I didn't think fasting applied to myself. I have a small body frame and I thought someone like me could not handle it. But during one of my visits to Siddhayatan I met a small-framed lady fasting for 30 days under Acharya Shree's guidance, and that's when I finally considered fasting. When you see others doing something, it shows there is a possibility for yourself too. I completed my first 24-hour water-only fast during another visit. Siddhayatan was the perfect place to do it, and Acharya Shree's guidance gave me the comfort I needed to know that everything would be okay. Surprisingly, my fast went fine and my body handled it pretty well. But the next day I was ready to eat!

When you fast, you experience as much as you allow yourself to experience. And when you go deep into the experience you can realize many things. I've realized that many of us are so fortunate to have access to food and water whenever we want it, things we so easily take for granted. I have realized that our human spirit is stronger than we think and that we can develop powers and unlock qualities hidden in our soul. I've also realized what people living in poverty might feel when they have nothing to eat. We lack humanity, and when we get a taste of some of the experiences of others it changes you inside. You see them and the world differently, you gain a sense of compassion and understanding for others and their pain.

I moved to Siddhayatan in 2013. Since then, I have done many fasts under Acharya Shree's guidance and supervision. I do water fasting, dry fasting, fruit fasting, or one meal per day (*ekasana*) with dry fasting between meals. For me, fasting is never easy, but the benefits I experience after are always far greater than the difficulties I face. All difficulties are worth pushing through so as long as it is safe for the body to keep going. Fasting has helped me build discipline, feel more connected with my soul, be more in tune with my physical body, stay healthy, and feel my body and mind becoming lighter – and that feeling is priceless.

During the years I have lived at Siddhayatan, I have seen Acharya Shree guide hundreds of our water fasting guests. I have also witnessed many miracles. Many people have healed their bodies from sickness, and although they achieve their goal, I have observed regularly that most lack spiritual understanding. When a person lacks understanding of the spiritual dimension, they will not reap the full benefits that can be uncovered at that level. I said many farewells to so many of our guests happy to complete their fasts. Some had been curious enough to ask spiritual questions, but many I felt could have gained so much more had they known more about the spiritual aspect. I also recognized, that many people had a lot of misinformation, misconceptions, and even wrong ideas about fasting, especially for breaking the fast. And that is the WHY of this book. After seeing this firsthand, I felt it was important for Acharya Shree to write an in-depth book about fasting so people could fast and break the fast safely, and most important to gain a deeper meaning and spiritual understanding of fasting. You cannot force people to be spiritual or to seek spiritual understanding. It has to come from them. However, if a person is ready and wishes to experience something deeper, it is important to have a good resource to learn from. So, I felt moved to ask Acharya Shree if he could sit with me and answer my questions as well as the most frequently asked questions by guests and students at Siddhayatan.

Acharya Shree is an enlightened master whose wisdom doesn't come from a book or his many degrees. Although he's considered a scholar with his mastery of ancient scriptures and ancient languages such as Sanskrit and Prakrit, his two master's degrees, and a Ph.D. in Philosophy, his most important knowledge comes from his lived experiences and from having reached the highest state of consciousness. In this highest state of being, he has attained the ability to guide through *Samyag Darshan* (right vision), *Samyag Jnana* (right knowing), and *Samyag Charitra* (right conduct). His extensive experience with fasting started many lives ago when he was living as a yogi in the most remote and fascinating areas of the Himalayas. He has guided thousands of people to fast safely following the ancient teachings of the Samanic Tradition.

In this book, Acharya Shree expands on the many aspects of spirituality and fasting. He answers all questions in a comprehensive and thought-out way, not from a scientific viewpoint, but rather from his immense inner knowing that only a master can do. This book will take you beyond the superficial fads of fasting, allowing you to experience purification from the deepest level of your being. Acharya Shree focuses on the purest of paths as described in the Dashvaikalik Sutra:

Dhammo Mangala Mukkitham, Ahimsa Sanjamo Tavo, Deva Vittam

Namam Santi, Jassa Dhame Saya Mano. "The three-folded path of non-violence, discipline, and austerity is the best and most auspicious path. Those whose mind is always on this path, even the angels will bow to them."

The teachings in this book bring blessings and transformation. I am beyond thrilled that you will get to learn the ancient origins of fasting, the connection between your mind, body, and soul through fasting, the impact of purification, the abundance of karma you can get rid of, and how you can practically liberate yourself by fasting. I hope that every person who reads this book gains spiritual understanding about fasting. I hope that everyone reaches their highest spiritual potential, and fortunately, we are blessed to have an enlightened master like Acharya Shree, to teach us a way to liberate our souls.

- Sadhvi Anubhuti

PART I:

FASTING FUNDAMENTALS

CHAPTER 1

INTRODUCTION TO FASTING

Fasting is the voluntary process of going without food, water, or both. Some people fast to heal their bodies, others to lose weight, and some to cleanse, and when you fast with those ideas that is all you get. However, those who fast for spiritual reasons will experience both health and spiritual benefits.

In general, when people think of fasting, they think of not eating, skipping meals, or giving up a food type. Some think that fasting is a form of starvation. Unfortunately, most people have limited knowledge about this ancient practice. In reality, fasting has been used for thousands of years as a spiritual practice, which has strengthened, awakened, purified, and uplifted spiritual practitioners.

Most people use fasting to heal and as a natural method to cure illness in their sick bodies. However, when people lack understanding of this practice, whether they do it for spiritual or health reasons, they can damage their bodies or not reap the full benefits of fasting.

Understanding fasting is critical when you use it as a spiritual practice. All spiritual practices need to be understood before practicing them. Guidance from those who have actually gone through the experience of fasting is of utmost importance. I have practiced fasting for over 50 years and have guided many in their fast. Many doctors or authors write books about fasting, but many have not even gone through the full experience themselves.

In this book, I will go into detail about the most important aspects of fasting so you can understand how you can use this practice to heal yourself, transform, burn your karma, and liberate your soul. Liberating your soul should be your ultimate goal in life. Every time you fast, you are stepping forward to achieving this goal. But first, you need to understand how fasting works and how it can help you achieve your goal.

Fasting is an English word, but in Sanskrit, there are multiple words for fasting. We call fasting *vrata*, *upavaasa*, *tapasya*, *tapashcharya*, and *tapa*. The words tapa, tapasya, and tapashcharya mean "fire." Fasting is a fire and it can burn many things. This fire can even burn karma, but it's important to not be confused about karma. People think karma results from good and bad deeds. No. Karma encompasses many aspects such as ignorance, illusion, anger, ego, hatred, jealousy, hallucinations, negativities, violence, and emotions. In one word, we call them karma, and they make our lives miserable. They make us suffer. Fasting is a fire that mostly burns karma. When karma disappears, illusion, hallucinations, and ignorance disappear too. When this happens, clarity comes naturally.

The most popular word we use in Sanskrit for fasting is tapa. Tapa means you make your body hot. The question is, how do we make our body hot? The answer is to not eat or drink anything, not even water. When you do this, the body inside becomes hot. As soon as the body becomes hot, it begins to burn. In the Upanishads, an ancient holy text that originally belonged to the Samanic and Jain traditions and now belongs to the Hindu Vedas, you can find the line "Tapasa Chiyate Brahma" or "through fasting you can achieve godhood." It is a proverb because fasting is difficult to do. People are addicted to alcohol, drugs, smoking, gambling, pornography, and other bad habits, but the most acute and terrible addiction is food, and when you fast, you have to drop that food. Whoever can give up food is the bravest person in the world, because dropping food is difficult. Usually, people give up food because doctors tell them to or because they are sick and can't eat. When something is wrong in your body and you cannot eat, it is not considered tapasya - a true fast.

When you have the flu, a fever, or your body cannot digest food because of sickness, and you cannot eat, that is not your choice. When sick, people can stay without eating for up to six months. That is not considered tapasya. Tapasya is very strange. Tapasya is the voluntary act of withdrawing yourself from eating. You decide out of the blue sky you will not eat or drink. Remember tapa is a fire, and tapasya is an austerity - you can do different types of tapasyas like eating only once a day, which also creates fire. The continuation of the fast is called tapashcharya, and there are many categories of this continuation.

The most popular word for fasting in India among Hindus is vrata. Vrata is like a vow. You take some vow to experience abstinence of food for a certain length of time. They may still drink water, tea, or juice but will not eat food. Some vratas can be very strict in the Hindu culture, like taking a vow to not eat or drink anything, not even water. It happens once a year during the Hindu holy day of *Nirjala Ekadashi* during the Hindu month of *Jyestha*. People observe an absolute or waterless fast on this day, which is challenging to do as it coincides with the hot Indian summer, making it a pious austerity. That is called vrata. When you take this vow wholeheartedly, you will stick to it no matter what.

The most significant and noteworthy word for tapasya, tapa, tapashcharya, or fasting is found in the Jain religion. In Jainism, they call it "upavaasa." It is the best word that represents these three. "Upa" means "near" and "vaasa" means "to live or reside." To live near your soul - your own spirit or consciousness. When you live near your consciousness, you enter into it, and when you do, you enjoy it. When you enter your consciousness, you close your senses. When you close your senses, you are not giving them food; your tongue wants to taste appetizing food, your nose wants to smell pleasing aromas, your eyes want to see what kind of dessert there is, or your ears want to hear flattering words. Upavaasa means you close all your senses, like a tortoise, when it sees danger and it withdraws its legs inside the shell. In the same way, in the real upavaasa, you pull all the senses, and they become closed inside, and when the senses are closed, they do not bother you. Why? Because you are doing it voluntarily. You go inside, and when you are inside, you live with your consciousness. Upavaasa means you live close to your soul. When a person lives close to their soul, they forget all the things that stimulate their senses.

I like upavaasa to describe tapa, tapasya, and tapashcharya the most as it encompasses the best representation of the time you spend while fasting. In English, we call it a fast, and in fasting, you can decide how many hours you wish to do it. Usually, one upavaasa or one vrata consists of 24 hours. You voluntarily choose not to eat or drink, or you may elect to abstain from eating or drinking select things. In the Samanic tradition, one upavaasa is considered almost 36 hours or sometimes even more. Why? Because they do not eat at night, so they practically fast for two nights and one day.

Understand that upavaasa has nothing to do with food; therefore, fasting has nothing to do with food. It is you going close to your soul, and when you go so close to your soul, you forget everything, including food. There are many ways to get close to your soul and live there. It can happen in many forms. I have witnessed people feel so close to their souls when they do something they genuinely enjoy.

For example, some people love listening to music, and if they listen wholly, they might forget to eat lunch or dinner because they are so into it. That music gives them happiness and joy in their heart – and the heart is the closest thing to the soul. Some people love reading novels or watching a series, and they forget about food and have no clue how much time has passed. This, too, can be considered upavaasa. When they naturally forget to eat, it is regarded as the best upavaasa. If the novel or movie is provoking the senses, then it is not considered upavaasa; however, if they are reading a book like *Siddhartha*, a story about the spiritual journey of self-discovery of a man named Siddhartha, then they are getting closer and closer to their soul or consciousness. When you live close to your consciousness and remember nothing, such as food or drinking, it means you are enjoying that mood, which allows you to go inside. When you fast, you strive to be in this mood, making your fast upavaasa -- residing close to your soul.

Upavaasa is the real fast. In the Jain tradition, upavaasa happens once a year during the auspicious celebration of *Paryushan* during August or September. Paryushan is a special celebration for 8-18 days if you consider both Jain traditions, *Svetambar* and *Digambar*. For 18 days, people read and learn how to improve themselves, obtain bliss in their soul, be awakened, and burn all their karma. They read books or spend time learning directly from the nuns and monks. It means they are doing upavaasa because they are in the mood to burn their karma and awaken their souls, and it happens naturally. It usually helps when people do this together. In India, Jain people get together and sit in front of monks and nuns asking them questions, and because the monks and nuns are not eating, they naturally do not eat. So, everyone enters this spiritual and uplifting mood.

Collectively, hundreds of thousands of people go in that direction. They are not only burning their karma, ignorance, clouds, and darkness, but they also obtain a lot of clarity. Once clarity comes to you, your soul cannot drown in the ocean of suffering. The soul gets dragged into the ocean of suffering because of the karmas you've collected. The best way to burn this karma is through upavaasa. Tapa and tapasya burn, but not as much as upavaasa. If you are ever in the mood to know or improve yourself, read those kinds of books, or talk to the monks and nuns, let it happen naturally. In general, this is the reason upavaasa is the best word for fasting.

One does upavaasa for spiritual reasons. If people do real upavaasa or fasting, no matter what has happened in their life in the past, their soul awakens. Their soul is like the sun rising high and coming out of the darkness. The soul comes out of the clouds, ignorance, and illusion. You do upavaasa, and it happens naturally. It occurs when you are wholeheartedly into it. Sometimes I give a lecture, and my students don't realize how much time has passed. They have expressed that one hour feels like five minutes. Why? Because they are in that mood, they listen and try to learn how to improve themselves or listen to their inner selves, what we call soul. And the real purpose of fasting is supposed to be that. The real purpose of fasting is to connect with yourself. To be with yourself. And that kind of fasting is the real thing. It takes you inside and makes you forget everything from the outside, including food, and that burns all of your karmas.

CHAPTER 2

ORIGINS OF FASTING

The history of fasting is very revolutionary. There is no historical time for its beginning. Our written history only goes back to five or ten thousand years. However, that is not enough information because fasting started when the planet formed millions of years ago. Historians and scientists believe that when the earth formed, it was like a fireball. It was scorching because the sun's proximity was closer, and there was almost no oxygen; therefore, there was no population or anything that could grow. It is believed that some humans survived inside the caves where the temperatures were somewhat tolerable. After thousands of years, the planet cooled down.

Most ancient civilizations, such as the Egyptian, Mayan, Chinese, or Mesopotamian do not mention the beginning of fasting in their cultures. One civilization that gives us a general idea about how fasting began is the Sindhu civilization. History is strange. I do not believe in history. Why? Because history is a lie. History is not true. It is incomplete. There are many aspects and angles to the truth, and the narrative of history is one-sided, so it misses many things. But when you go deep into your meditative state, you get the facts. There you find the reality.

When this planet cooled down, the first clouds and moisture formed. The few humans who had survived and lived in caves came out for the first time. It was still boiling during the day, but they would come out at night to watch and feel the coolness the moon created. For their initial survival, they would go to the riverbanks to fish and do other things at night. Later, the rain began. It rained continuously for seven weeks, and this rain continued to cool down the earth until vegetation grew. At first, the cavemen feared what was growing as they had never seen greenery or anything like it. Quickly, plants, bushes, and flora grew. Certain types of vegetation can develop within a short period, and this was seven weeks, which allowed many plants to grow. The cavemen would touch the plants at night, and they realized that they were harmless, so they tasted them. In a few weeks, some plants grew fruits, like berries. They tasted them and realized they were sweet and not like meat. The meat was different, which is what they were accustomed to eating. The new weather, coolness, and vegetation had started, and this made the cavemen very happy. Everyone from the caves came out and realized that the foliage was so beautiful and did not hurt or kill them. They thought it was sweet and better than meat.

The revolutionary step took place on the 49th day after the rain stopped. They thought, "Whatever this superpower is, which is controlling us, whether it is nature or something else, it has given us the idea to drop the meat." On this day, they decided that because now they had different things to eat, that they would not eat meat anymore. They thought they would now be vegetarian and only eat what nature was giving them, like fruits, berries, etc. It was the first revolutionary step in human history, and to celebrate this day, they thought, "Why don't we stop eating and drinking for one day?" It was the start of fasting. The first notion of fasting concerned this celebration. A celebration that God or nature had given them this vegetation, which tasted much better than anything they had tasted before. They gathered to talk about it all day, and they were so into it because it was a wonder; it was something never seen or experienced before. This day is what I call the revolutionary step in human history. Most people have forgotten about this step, but I haven't.

Fasting, from a historical viewpoint, started with dry fasting, not even water. I call this the first step. The cavemen had no idea why they were doing it, but they were doing it as a transition from meat-eating to vegetarianism, and for this transition, they wanted to celebrate. How did they celebrate? Dancing? No. They celebrated by fasting for at least one day by not putting anything in their mouth. The birth of fasting was a dry fast. Today, you can see the lasting influence of this celebration. In Hindu culture, dry fasting happens one day a year by tradition. Even though they are in India, they are forgetting this tradition in the Hindu culture. They do it only for one day. Maybe that one day is the one day that represents the historic step.

But the Samanic Jain tradition is predominantly keeping dry fasting alive; they dry fast at least one to ten days each year. The Samanic tradition still carries the tradition to dry fast, and they do it at least once a year. Most monks, nuns, *shravaks* and *shravikas* (male and female householders, respectively), dry fast during this time. They call this time *Samvatsari*, which means "after one year one day." They not only fast, but they have also added one extra step. They want to experience what monkhood is like, so for one day, they visit the monks and spend the full day with them, participating in the same activities the monks engage in. The men go with the monks and the women with the nuns. They fast together and hear *pravachans*, spiritual lectures, from them. Like the monks, the laypeople sleep on the floor very simply; it doesn't matter if they are rich people, millionaires, or billionaires; they wear the monk clothes and spend time with them while dry fasting. The Jain tradition added one revolutionary step, which is to experience monkhood while dry fasting.

Initially, the cavemen did not know it would burn karma. They had little understanding about anything. They did it as a celebration because it was a new thing, and for them to be without food and water was a big step. I call it a stepping stone in fasting history, which, unfortunately, other countries do not carry this message. They have an idea of fasting, but they do not have the pure concept of fasting. From a health viewpoint, we are seeing that some people have begun to dry fast. In the U.S.A., they have tough and strict laws, and if they know someone is teaching about dry fasting and something happens, they can get in a lot of trouble. But in countries like Russia, they do dry fasting for up to 10 days for health reasons, and without many restrictions. They have no idea about karma. Later I will discuss how fasting burns all the karma, and once karma is destroyed, your soul becomes clear and pure. The cavemen started fasting, but the Samanic tradition added the concept of fasting to burn karma.

When the Samanic people carried this idea of dry fasting, they noticed that their bodies became so light. Their head became light and they experienced something much deeper internally. As they realized how fasting made their bodies and senses feel, they understood that fasting was the cause. Hence, fasting began for spiritual reasons.

How does fasting in the old period compare to today?

In the past, fasting was very challenging. When people would fast, for them, it meant everything was fully closed. They would not brush their teeth or use water to clean themselves because they wanted to be entirely out of the water, even by touch. They thought, why bother with those things if it's only for a few days? Their idea was to use their body to create a fire that would burn their karma. They believed that if they kept cleaning the body, their senses would get stronger. They intended to make the senses entirely weak as to not tempt one to taste, see, smell, or hear things that would stimulate the senses. Their theory was that they would bring the senses inward, like a turtle when it brings its legs inside to protect itself. These days, people still brush their teeth, clean themselves, shower, wear nice clothes during their fast, and in a way, it is good because they are fasting only one day here and there. But in the old time, there were no clothes. There was no cloth industry; they only wore leaves they would wrap around their body like the native people still do. There were no showers, they used to bathe in the river, but they would not go during the fast because their idea was to protect all living beings in the bodies of water and not enchant their senses. They did not want to give food or strength to the senses.

The more food you give to the senses, the stronger they become. The same applies to the mind. If you feed the mind, the stronger it gets. What is the food for the mind? Food for the mind is what the mind likes, and it wants to hear pleasant words, enjoyable music, and a good conversation that stimulates it. When one is in the mind, they are not in the soul. In the old days, external stimulation was forbidden during fasting. They would only talk about the soul. They would only engage in spiritual conversations about how to go beyond the mind and the senses. It is the reason, in the old days, fasting was the most difficult. Even though they were not very knowledgeable, they were intuitively using their body as an instrument and would burn more karma than us. Why? Not only because they had a more robust body than us, but also, they were so disciplined to not cross to the other side at all. The other side means the side that feeds the senses and mind.

When people would do something, they were indulged into it. They did not have as many distractions, so if they would fast, they would burn karma. If they meditated, they were fully immersed in meditating. In this aspect, they used to burn a lot of karma. But even though they used to burn more karma than us, because they were more into it, the current human body has the ability to burn even more karma than in the past. Physically speaking, what we go through nowadays is a lot more intense because when we fast, we get weak, dizzy, sick, nauseous, and this creates chaos in the body, especially during extended fasting. It automatically puts you in that kind of suffering and pain, and it is all voluntary. No one makes you do it, and the body can suffer for five, six, or seven days, depending on each person's body. We now can burn more karma because our body structure is very frail. Throughout the different periods of the planet, there are six human body structures, and we have the last one -- the weakest one. It is the weakest structure, and it creates a lot of chaos when we stop eating or drinking water. When this happens, it invites your karma to surface so that you can burn it. Suppose a particular karma was supposed to give you a result in one hundred lives; when you fast, you invite it so you can burn it quicker and a lot sooner. Can you believe that with this weakest structure, if you fast for only one day, it equals 30 days of fasting during Tirthankara Mahavira's time? This was over 2,600 years ago.

The weakest structure can burn the most karma when fasting. It burns an abundance of karma, mountain-high karma like the tallest mountain in the world, Mt. Everest. It is difficult to destroy it, but it is possible. Fasting makes it so. Right now, is the luckiest time to be on this earth. Hindus ignorantly perceive this as the worst period, and they call it Kali Yuga. I tell them this is the best time. Kali Yuga does not mean the worst time. It means it is the era of machinery. "Kal" in Sanskrit means "machine." It means we have technology, and we have everything. They have misunderstood and misinterpreted the concept of Kali Yuga. Then there is Maha Kali Yuga, which they believe to be much worse, similar to an apocalypse. They believe people will suffer a lot, which creates a massive fear because they envision this dreadful time is on its way. But it is not true. It just means there will be even more technology. Yes, I agree that people will be too much into technology and it will create a lot of problems, but it doesn't mean it is a bad period. It is the best period if you understand that even if you do something small for your spiritual upliftment, it will bring you a significant result. The more you can do to grow spiritually, the more you will benefit from this era.

Kali Yuga is the best period and I consider Maha Kali Yuga to be even better. The best of best. Why? The body will get weaker and weaker, and if someone gets on the spiritual path and follows it, they will burn a lot more karma. If they are not on the path, it is a different story, but if they are, they can burn a lot of karma, and they can go faster towards liberation. For some, it could take many lives or thousands of years, so it is best to take advantage of these two crucial periods while you can.

How do body types differ between now and then?

As I mentioned earlier, there are six structures of the human body. In the past, the bodies of extraordinary individuals, such as Tirthankara Mahavira, were exceptionally strong. The name of their body type is *vajra rushabha naracha sanhanana* which translates to "adamantine nerves, joints, and bone formations." *Vajra* means stone - a unique stone that cannot break. A vajra diamond is so strong that if you place it on top of a solid iron shield and hammer it, it will dent it and go inside the iron instead of breaking. Bodies, like the one Tirthankara Mahavira had, are like that; their bones cannot break. So, if this type of body fasts for one day, they burn very little karma. If they fast for 30 days, then they will burn a lot of karma. But presently, the structure of the human body is fragile. Our body type is called *sevartak* or *asamprapta strupatica sanhanana*, which means "that the skin holds our bones, and there is not much to keep them together." Our shoulders, hips, ankles, or any joint can easily dislocate from an injury, and without help from an expert, it is difficult to put them back in place. This can create tremendous pain and even immobilize you.

Other structures were different, and they were connected differently; also, they never suffered from dislocations. Our current structure is considered the weakest. I would not consider this a disadvantage, though. Remember, if you fast for only one day, you will benefit tremendously. It means we have more chances to burn karma. The big question in all this is: Do we have a pure mind when we fast? If we have a pure mind, then yes, we can burn a lot of karma in one day. But if you are fasting for health reasons, as most people do, or for weight loss, then the idea is to get rid of fat and not karma. Such intentions don't burn karma, that is why when you fast you should check your intention. Is it to burn fat or to burn karma? If you intend to burn fat, your soul will not wake up. Why? Because you are burning fat due to you wanting to look beautiful or slim - you want to be good-looking in society. There are advantages to all body structures. However, we are blessed to have today's body constitution as an instrument to burn all of our karma.

To briefly describe the six structures per the Samanic tradition, there is the strongest structure, which I described earlier. That is the vraja rushabha naracha sanhanan and it has adamantine nerves, joints, and bone formations. The *vraja naracha sanhanana* structure has adamantine joints and bone formations. The *naracha sanhanana* structure has unbreakable joints and bones formations. The *ardha narach sanhanana* structure has semi-unbreakable joints and bones formations. The *kilika sanhanana* structure has rived bones formations. And lastly, which is the current body structure we have, asamprapta strupatica sanhanana, which has loosely joined bones formations. The type of body we have not only depends on this time period, but also your karma.

Who realized that fasting burns karma?

The cavemen nor the first people in the Samanic tradition knew that fasting burned karma. The realization of this process happened when the first extraordinary person was born. His name was Adinath, the first enlightened master and first *Tirthankara*. We also call him Adi Baba or Adishwar Baba. *Adi* means" first", and *Baba* means "enlightened one." It somehow got twisted in Hindu culture; some people still call him Adinath or Adi Baba, but mostly he became known as Shiva. Many scholars and devotees ignore that Tirthankara Adinath was the pioneer to teach about fasting for spiritual reasons.

He taught that fasting burns karma and illusion and that it brings purity and clarity. The first Tirthankara was the first one to teach about this.

You may wonder who a Tirthankara is. In the Samanic tradition, a Tirthankara is an extraordinary person in the world. They were born with three kinds of knowledge: *Mati Gyan or* super intelligence, *Shrut Gyan* or knowledge which comes by hearing, and *Avadhi Gyan* or telescopic vision. Later in their life, they explore and attain two more types of knowledge called *Manahparyaya Gyan* and *Keval Gyan*. Manahparyaya Gyan is the ability to read the particles of a developed mind, and Keval Gyan is absolute knowledge, also known as enlightenment. They embody the purest virtues, such as non-violence, forgiveness, truthfulness, and compassion, and dedicate their lives to the earnest search of truth in the universe. The path they walk is the most difficult path, taking complete responsibility for their lives and living according to the highest spiritual principles to dissolve their karma and reach enlightenment, liberating themselves from the cycle of ignorance, pain, suffering, birth, and death.

Tirthankaras are little known outside of India today, though their teachings have unknowingly affected millions of people worldwide. Tirthankara is a Sanskrit word meaning "one who makes the harbor." Why make a harbor? To cross the ocean, you need to get on a ship, and to get on the ship, you must find the harbor. Around the Tirthankara, the *Tirtha* is formed. Tirtha is the harbor, the home of the ship. So, the figurative meaning is the ocean of suffering, ocean of pain, and we need to cross it. If we have the right teachings, then the crossing becomes possible; otherwise, we'll wander here and there, maybe going in the wrong direction. You can also say God; without God, you cannot go further, and a Tirthankara is like a living God. They are an extraordinary type of enlightened master. Even the few enlightened masters on this earth today are not Tirthankaras. They are rare and exceptional. You can ask them questions and they will guide you through your path and help you to raise your consciousness to the highest state. Without a body, God cannot communicate.

In our time cycle, there were 24 Tirthankaras, and they all experienced incredible suffering, which is why they had a unique body. Their body was very strong and had a structure different from ours. It was so strong that even if someone with a modern gun attacked them, the bullets would not penetrate their skin. Whatever happens to a Tirthankara's body while they're alive will not kill them. This is why I say that Tirthankaras are extraordinary – they are a kind of super-human. They can tolerate so much, but they remain balanced and unaffected throughout their suffering because they know that whatever is happening to them is just the result of their karma; they brought it on themselves from their past lives. There is at least 70 Tirthankaras and a maximum of 120 Tirthankaras in the universe. They are accessible to help you via deep meditation. On this earth, in this era, the last Tirthankara was Tirthankara Mahavira.

Historically speaking, Tirthankara Adinath is beyond history. He was the first Tirthankara and the ruler of the early Indian civilization. His statue was found in sitting meditation position, and his teachings were popular among the first civilization of the Sindhu era, which is at least 8,000 years old, historically. If his teachings were widespread during that time, it means he could have been born 100,000 years ago or more. So, he is not a historical figure; he is prehistoric like the caveman.

Tirthankara Adinath renounced his kingdom to become an ascetic to focus on the inner journey to liberate his soul. He acknowledged that society those days was carrying a marvelous tradition to fast and he taught them that fasting was a tool to burn karma. It was only until then that the definition of fasting was refined, and it was understood how it could burn karma when doing upavaasa. He polished many other things, but he was the leader who taught that fasting burns karma. He taught and led based on his own experiences and realizations. For a couple of decades, he did a lot of tapasya or upavaasa. He would sit in meditative state for up to eight days without moving, eating, or drinking water. Most of his followers left him because they could not keep up with his pace of not even drinking water. But his body was so impressively strong that he kept doing it until after a couple of decades, he reached his goal and enlightenment entered his body. After enlightenment, he began to teach. The real karmic theory on how to burn it by fasting, tapasya, or upavaasa originated with the first Tirthankara.

Tirthankara Adinath became the first yogi, and there is no trace of his exact lifetime period. What's interesting is popular yogis, scholars, and gurus are not even aware of this truth. But some people who portray themselves as *sadhgurus* or "true gurus" claim that

Tirthankara Adinath, also known as *Adi Yogi*, was born 15,000 years ago. But they are not knowledgeable, and they have no idea. The reality is gone. Many Hindu *swamis*, also known as renunciants, lack knowledge about what they are talking about, and even though I come from the same tradition, I condemn those people in this aspect. Why? Because they lack knowledge, and they misinform people. They need to go deep into their own consciousness or enlightenment to know that they cannot predict Tirthankara Adinath's exact period. If they are not enlightened, they can go deep into a meditative state to reflect and have some light that makes them realize that Adi Yogi did not exist 15,000 years ago. Recorded history goes back to 10,000 years, and some cave paintings go back to maybe 40,000 years ago. If someone had a picture or statue 15,000 years ago, perhaps the figure is that many years old, but it does not mean that the person carved in the stone lived during that time. Instead, it could have been millions of years ago.

The Samanic tradition originated the yogic system, and the Samanic tradition was started by Tirthankara Adinath. His name can still be found throughout history and in the major religions. In Hindu culture, he's also known as Adinath. In Islam, he is called Adam Baba. He was also really popular in Africa. If you go to Ethiopia, a heavily Christian and Muslim populated country, you will find out that the capital is called Addis Ababa after his name. His name traveled to every continent, and by the time it reached the west, it became Adam. But he is the same person. Adam means "the first one," and he was the first enlightened one and the first to introduce the teachings of burning karma. All of the Tirthankaras carry the teachings of burning karma. Even if there is a big gap between them of hundreds of thousands of years, they still hold the same idea and message.

What were the fasting experiences of the Tirthankaras?

As you now know, the first Tirthankara was Adinath. His symbol is the bull. Every Tirthankara has a symbol that represents the society in which they lived. The society during his time was very innocent and pure. The bull is a very good animal, which carries the bullock cart's weight without hesitation. Even if the bull is thirsty, they will not sit on the way and will take the load to the destination. Other animals do not do that. Horses will not go further unless you give them water. That is why Tirthankara Adinath's society's symbol is the bull because it represents the society of those days: resilient, innocent, and pure.

Tirthankara Adinath's body was remarkable. His body was like Tirthankara Mahavira's -- indestructible with conspicuous strength. One time he fasted for almost one year. He took a vow that he would not break the fast unless he received something specific, sugarcane juice. After taking the vow, he went into silence, so he couldn't talk to anyone. Inevitably, people offered him things because he was considered the king of kings, so they would offer him diamonds, clothes, gold, jewelry, but no one offered him food. No one knew what to do. They thought he was a king, so they didn't know what to offer him, and they did not know that he could not ask for food. He finally went to Hastinapur, near Delhi, where his grandson was ruling. His grandson came to see him and brought him sugarcane juice. It was the first time anyone had offered it to him, so he broke his fast after almost one year. His body survived, but if we think our body can also survive in the same way, we are wrong. Our body would break down. It would die. Tirthankara Adinath had the strength and the strongest body to do this type of prolonged fasting, and so did his son Gommateshwara, also known as Bahubali. Bahubali fasted for one year in a standing meditative pose. The karma they used to burn in one year is what we comparatively burn in only 12 days.

Tirthankara Mahavira dry fasted for almost six months, five months and 27 days, to be exact. However, Tirthankara Mahavira's soul was indisputably surrounded by too much karma. It is said that if you combined the karma of all the other 23 Tirthankaras, he had even more than that. He had to go through a lot of suffering, but he was so brave and that is why we call him Mahavira, which means "the bravest one." His real name was Vardhamana and he was the 24th and last Tirthankara to be born on this planet, which was over 2,600 years ago. He taught us so much about perseverance on the spiritual path.

When you recognize there are different body types, even today, it helps to understand that we cannot compare ourselves when we fast. Fasting has to go according to each person's body. It is best neither to compare or compete. Remember that we carry the weakest structure, and even if we do a little bit of fasting, it gives you a significant result.

One thing to know is that with this weak structure we have, if a person does the worst thing in the world, they cannot collect the heaviest karma that takes them to the worst hellish planet. There are seven hellish planets, the seventh one being the worst, where the most extreme misery and suffering occur. With our current structure, the maximum they will reach is the first hellish planet, which is not as terrible. But this body cannot collect that much or that kind of karma to take you to the seventh hellish planet. Likewise, people cannot enjoy that much with this body structure. When you have the stronger structures like Tirthankaras, you collect too much karma when you enjoy something too much. Thus, consider this current structure a blessing that gives you a good result if you do something good, even if it is a little. The best time for spiritual growth, transformation, and liberation is now.

CHAPTER 3

RELIGION & FASTING

The most popular religions and philosophies in the world practice fasting for different lengths of time, purposes, and outcomes. Jainism, Buddhism, Christianity, Islam, Judaism, Taoism, and Hinduism are among the common groups that take on fasting for different purposes, but commonly for penance and sacrifice. Though they are doing it for penance and sacrifice, most lack the concept of karma, which misses a profound spiritual element to fasting. What they do know is that after fasting, they feel good. But if they have no idea of the fundamental concept to burn karma, they will never be in that mood, thinking, or state of burning their karma.

Jainism

Presently, Jainism is the only religion that teaches in-depth the concept of burning karma while fasting. In Jainism, fasting is not an obligation; instead, it is a voluntary endeavor to awaken and free the soul.

The Jain religion comes from the Samanic tradition, and the Samanic tradition started with Tirthankara Adinath. The term "Jain" did not exist in those days, but Jainism is currently one of the last and most popular branches of the Samanic tradition. Jain means "follower of the Jinas," and Jinas are those who have won victory over themselves – they have gone beyond hatred and attachment. Jains still follow the same ideas of fasting. Each year, they fast on water for at least eight days during Paryushan, but they have many types of fasts they follow throughout the year according to their bodies' ability.

There is a saying in the Jain religion, "You can fast every day if you eat one bread less than your hunger." Eating less is also fasting. They rarely do juice fasting because they believe that fruits and raw vegetables carry many germs, so they think it is better not to do it. They may do *Ekasana* fasting, eating one meal once a day while sitting in one position. Once you are seated, you cannot move from there. Another fast they practice is called *Ayambil*, a much more difficult fast that burns even more karma than water fasting. Traditionally, Ayambil is eating a wheat-like grain once a day. You cook it with no oil, ghee, butter, salt, spices, or anything else. You eat it plain. It is like bread, and in the real Ayambil, you break the bread into pieces and you dip it into water. You let it get mushy and then you eat it only once during the day. There is no taste at all; this is Ayambil. When there is taste in the food, it means your senses are active. The best is when there is no taste in the food because then the senses go dormant. The principle behind it is to eliminate all the taste. And it is very difficult to eat that mushy food, you really do not want to eat it, but you are disciplining yourself. For this reason, you go beyond the dislike.

In a way, Ayambil is better than water fasting. Because it is hard to eat it. You know you don't like it because it is tasteless, but you know you have to eat. You eat one piece at a time. And this practice of discipline burns a lot of karma versus avoiding food and drinking water. The body is used to taste, taste, and taste, and that's why it becomes a problem.

Another common type of fast Jains do is called *Pahar Porsi*. You eat and drink after the first quarter of the day passes, about three hours after sunrise. Whatever builds up or accumulates in the body from overnight sleeping, you allow it to burn when you do not eat or drink anything for this period. It is a gentle way to fast, and people, in general, can do that much. It is not a big deal; every day, you can wait to eat after three hours from sunrise, and you'll benefit a lot.

I suggest that you do not eat or drink anything until after sunrise. In India, Jains wait at least 48 minutes after sunrise because that is how long it takes for the acid in the body to burn. It is a common practice that both householders and monks follow. In Jainism, they have many fasting variations, but most importantly, they fast for upavaasa. They forget everything as they close off their senses to be close to their soul in a meditative state and burn karma bondage, which keeps a soul away from liberation and bliss.

Hinduism

Hindus support a lot of fasting throughout the year. It is a very integral part of their culture. They fast for many reasons, from the purification of the soul to gaining something spiritual or materialistic. During the holy celebration of Nirjala Ekadashi, they abstain from eating food and drinking water, but few Hindus can do dry fasting. During Ram Navami, another holiday, they celebrate the birthday of Rama. To celebrate, they fast because they want to be pure like Rama. Rama is considered a god in Hindu culture, but in reality he was an enlightened one. During this celebration, they do not eat meats, grains, beans, or other heavy foods. They only drink juice and eat fruits, vegetables, or very light foods.

Navaratri is another important Hindu holiday where everyone fasts for ten days. They do a lot of prayer, meditation, go to the temple, listen to spiritual discourses, and don't fight or get angry. The environment becomes very spiritual. It happens throughout all of India, so it becomes a beautiful and positive time. I am talking about almost one billion people doing this together. That is the beauty of it. When one billion people do it collectively, it creates such beautiful energy. When people visit India during those days, they think India is a spiritual country because everyone is in that mood. Everyone is fruit fasting, enjoying, and growing spiritually. At the same time, they become healthier as their body cells regenerate, a byproduct of the fruit fasting.

Buddhism

Like Jains, Buddhists follow different forms of fasting. Among the nuns and monks, some stop eating after noon. As a form of fasting, some Buddhist traditions do not eat meats for a specific length of time. They also have a Nyungne fast, which is to eat vegetarian food one day, and on the second day, they refrain from both food and water. Like Jains, they may also practice Ekasana, eating one meal only, but they call it *Ekāsanikanga*. Buddhists used to have the concept of fasting to burn karma too, but nowadays, it seems like they are forgetting this teaching and fast more for the practice of self-control and self-discipline.

Christianity

In Christianity, it is not commanded to fast; however, many Christians fast throughout the year primarily by reducing their food intake during a predetermined time. In the Bible, there are many references to fasting. Some sects believe that God rewards fasting, and some do not encourage fasting as a way to solely rely on the belief of being saved by grace through their faith alone.

Christian denominations who observe Lent to commemorate the 40-day fast observed by Jesus during his temptation in the desert do a partial fast or give up something for 40 days. Currently, the emphasis to fast is set on Ash Wednesday and Good Friday when they abstain from eating meat, except for fish.

If you look at Catholicism, they have always supported fasting. In the early Catholic teachings, they even used to include the karma and reincarnation concepts. At present, though, the tradition to fast remains, but the concept is forgotten. Catholicism, in many ways, is an imitation of the Jain religion, not entirely but mostly. Christianity is a little over 2000 years old, Jainism or the Samanic Tradition, we do not know when it started, but historically it is at least 10,000 years old. Somehow, Catholics came into contact with the teachings, and they adopted fasting, but they forgot altogether the concept and theory behind it. They now do it to purify themselves, and they are purifying themselves for sure, but it does not mean they will burn the karma. They need to have the concept in their mind to burn the karma. This way, the senses cannot tempt them to break the fast in the middle.

Mormons fast the first Sunday of every month. They call it Fast Sunday, and they abstain from eating and drinking for two consecutive meals. They do it to worship God. In addition, whatever money they would have spent on eating that day, they donate it to their church to assist the poor and needy.

Many Seventh-day Adventists abstain from eating meats and follow a vegetarian or vegan diet as a way of living. They believe their body is holy and that they should only eat the healthiest foods. According to studies from Loma Linda University in California, Adventists who follow this lifestyle increase their life span up to ten years longer than those who do not follow their strict vegetarian principles.

If you travel to Africa, you might be surprised to find out that Christians in Egypt and Ethiopia fast for at least 180 days and up to 252 days each year. Their fasting involves not eating meat, eggs, or dairy products. For at least 180 days, they are not only vegetarian, they are vegan. Those who adhere to the strict guidelines only partake in one meal to be eaten in the afternoon or evening, and they do not eat or drink anything before 3:00 pm.

Judaism

Judaism is the oldest religion in the West. During their Yom Kippur holiday, they abstain from food and water for 25 hours. During the day, they pray, reflect, and repent from their sins. They have many other days when they fast for reparation of wrongdoing, mourning, gratitude, or commemoration.

Islam

Islam also supports fasting, and they call it *Sawm*. Muslims see fasting as a religious obligation during Ramadan and are mandated to abstain from food, drinks, smoking, and sexual activity between sunrise and sunset. They do exempt specific individuals from fasting, such as pregnant women or children. For one month, they take a fasting vow not to consume food or water during the day. They are dry fasting during the day. In Arab countries, this is very difficult because it is the summertime and the days are very hot and long.

Muslims are doing a remarkable thing by fasting during the day. However, there is a big drawback with the way and time they break the fast. When they break the fast, they have a big feast, and they eat too much food. If they only ate once, it would not be that big of a deal, but they wake up early in the morning and have another feast before the sunrise. This is the worst time to put food in the stomach. Why? Because our solar plexus, the navel, is directly interconnected with the sun. When the sun is not present, the solar plexus is fully closed. It works like a lotus flower; it closes at night and opens during the day. Until the solar plexus is not awake, the food does not get digested properly.

I advise you never to eat anything before your solar plexus opens. Your system is still asleep, it's closed off, and you are congesting it by putting food inside. But Muslims eat before sunrise. And I have seen that a lot of Muslim brothers and sisters gain weight during Ramadan. Why? Because they are filling up their stomach two times. I do not support this idea. This is counterproductive for their health. If they ate only one meal, it would be considered Ekasana, and they could still lose weight and improve their health.

Another downside is that in Islam, they have no concept of vegetarianism. At least they do not eat pork, but to break the fast, they pretty much eat anything they want. After breaking a 12-hour dry fast, you need to be very careful not to overeat or eat heavily toxic foods like meat; otherwise, it's detrimental to their health and it can create a lot of trouble. When breaking a fast, I suggest always eating light vegetarian food easy on the system and not damaging.

Muslims experience many other benefits while fasting. They pray a lot, avoid fighting, arguing, or lustful thoughts. They are in a good mood for one month, but they miss out on the karmic and health benefits. To benefit at the karmic level, you need to have the concept of karma. Most religions miss out on this level.

Whatever each person's idea is for fasting, it will only do that much. You need to know that you are fasting for your spiritual upliftment. Only then, your karma will burn.

CHAPTER 4

FASTING ESSENTIALS

Everyone knows that all machines must rest if they work for 24 hours. Cars, tractors, and trucks are all machines, and they all need rest. Likewise, the human body is a machine, and it is the most complex machine in the whole universe. The human machine has numerous parts and components, and they need rest too. If you do not give them rest, they will create a lot of trouble and pain. Because of our lack of knowledge, we invite a lot of diseases. We have created many terrible habits, especially with food. We indulge in excess, eat an abundance of junk food and things we cannot digest, ingest too much medicine, consume highly toxic drinks like wine or hard liquor, or heavily toxic foods like meats and processed foods. People love these things, and they become a slave to their taste, but it creates a lot of trouble in the body.

With these acquired bad habits, it is imperative to let our machine get rest. Even if you give it rest for one day, it might get a little better. It becomes like a tune-up. You tune up the car, so why not tune up your body, your machine? Unfortunately, people only tune it up when they get sick. Like when someone has a fever, they cannot eat. When a person cannot eat, it is your machine telling you, "Give me rest." But people do not understand these symptoms. And if you do not listen, your machine will overheat. When you get sick and cannot eat, it means you are putting too much into your body. Before it gives you trouble, give it a break and to let it rest. Trouble is when you experience blockages, disease, sickness, muscle pain, aches, calcium buildup, cancer, heart disease, arthritis, diabetes, and so many other things.

Humans only rest their bodies when they are sick and don't feel like eating. If you force them to eat, they will vomit. So, this is the only time they give their body a rest, which is not considered the real rest. Rest is when you do it voluntarily. You decide that you will give it rest for one full day, ideally at least once per month. And when you do, your body runs smoothly. If you usually eat less or eat light foods, your body will not need as much rest. But if you eat heavy, greasy, rich, and fried foods, then your body will need at least one day of rest per week. If you eat too much meat like pork, beef, or other meats, your body will need to rest twice a week because they are considered very heavy and toxic. So, it all depends on what you put into your body.

Some doctors will not understand this and may attack me because they think that if you do not eat, you will not survive, and that your muscles will get weak. They consider this body only as a combination of muscles, tissues, bones, organs, nervous system, etc. They see muscles are getting weak, but they don't see that the muscles are getting rest. Remember, you need to tune up your machinery. I'm not saying you have to fast too much. Anything over done and in excess is not good either. Our human body has a very weak structure, and it can break if you force it to fast too much, and people can die. It has happened in India, they forced themselves to fast too much and they died.

If your body is not feeling well, break the fast right away. It doesn't make you a weak person to break and end your fast early and that you cannot reach your personal goal. Practice non-violence towards your own body.

Even after three days, if you do not feel comfortable, break it. There is nothing wrong with that, you tried, and that is enough. Maybe your body only needed a three-day rest. So, don't push further. Your body will tell you when to break, and you need to listen.

How does the body clean itself while fasting?

From a science and health perspective, when you fast, the body needs to pull energy from something. If you feed the body food, juice, or some other sustenance, the body will draw energy from there.

When you water fast or dry fast, the body uses the stored glucose in the system, specifically in the liver. The glucose in the liver takes anywhere between 10 to 12 hours to burn. Once the body finishes using this glucose, it breaks down the excess glucose turned into fat. This is the point when people lose weight. It takes a long time to finish all the fat. This process is called ketosis, and during this process, the body also repairs itself.

During fasting, the body can recycle materials left in the intestines and the stomach rapidly, which cleans the digestive system. The harmful bacteria in the gut cease, and the good microbes reproduce. Damaged cells get repaired while old parts of the immune system get flushed out, and good cells regenerate. Toxins burn – fat burns. The body eats disease and cancerous cells. And this is how the body heals and regenerates itself. This process is called autophagy. All the organs, muscles, digestive system, blood, and all body parts get cleaned, repaired, and purified. For health and wellness, it is no surprise why fasting is becoming such a big trend throughout the world.

What are the common types of fasting?

From giving up your favorite food to the arduous experience of giving up all food and water, there are many forms, degrees, and lengths of fasting. The various fasts can help you achieve detoxification, emotional cleansing, mental clarity, self-discipline, improved health, resetting, spiritual upliftment, soul purification, and much more.

The body needs nourishment at all times. Nourishment means eating wholesome, healthy, light, and freshly cooked food. This food will provide balance, nutrition, and wellness. But because of our lack of knowledge, bad habits, or inability to eating healthy, we accumulate many toxins. When you fast, you burn all the toxins built up in your body. It is like changing the oil of a car. When the vehicle has burnt oil, the oil needs to be changed; otherwise, the car will no longer function. Once you drain it and put new oil, the car runs a lot smoother. In the same way, when you practice certain fasts like juice fasting, water fasting, or dry fasting, it is like changing the oil from your body. And what is the burnt oil in the body? Toxins. And toxins are sitting all over the body. We've collected many toxins by putting heavily toxic foods in our system like meats, canned, fried, and processed foods.

These fasts are the most common forms of fasting. Each type of fast can have variations, and the benefits will change according to the type, length, intention, and how much you are into it.

Juice fasting

Juice fasting takes toxins out of your body. The juice has to be made fresh and only a few minutes before drinking it for optimal results. I strongly do not recommend store-bought or bottled juice. These juices have preservatives or may have sat on the shelf for long periods. After only 30 minutes of making fresh juice, the oxidation process begins. Oxidation is the process that makes the juice lose its nutritional value, so the sooner you drink the juice, the better.

Also, know that juice fasting involves drinking limited amounts of juice. Limited means no more than 16 ounces, maybe twice a day. You need to gain knowledge of proper combinations of fruits and vegetables. Sometimes certain fruits don't go together, or some fruits don't go with certain vegetables. If done correctly, juice fasting helps to attack toxins and rebuild new cells in the body. Fresh juices can have carrots, celery, beet, ginger, berries, apples, kale, and many other fruits and vegetables. Before you start, it is essential to research what combinations go together before mixing many ingredients.

Pros: It will help gently detox the body. Your body receives nourishment from all the nutrients the fruits and vegetables carry.
Cons: If fruits and vegetables are not appropriately cleaned, harmful bacteria can enter the body. The wrong combination of juices can damage the body's system.

Water Fasting

When you do water fasting for 24 - 36 hours, it will drain many more toxins than juice fasting. Those who genuinely wish to improve their health and cleanse their body need to drink water only. Some people add vitamins, minerals, salt, or supplements to the water, but this is not as effective as keeping the fast pure with only water. When fasting, sickness in the body vanishes because the toxins are the ones making the person sick. If the toxins decrease, a person doesn't get sick, and health improves. Toxins always build up, hence the importance of water fasting regularly. When you water fast, you give your body a full break because it doesn't have to process anything for digestion. The body never gets rest unless you stop to fast. When the body gets a break, the organs, muscles, tissues, and digestive system all get a break too.

Pros: When you water fast for one day, you get the health benefits of a 4-day juice fast. Water fasting burns more toxins.
Cons: If your body has a lot of acidity, if you consume too much caffeine, or eat an unhealthy diet, water fasting will be challenging initially.

Dry Fasting

Abstaining from food and fluid is dry fasting. Dry fasting drains a lot more toxins because dry fasting creates a bigger fire in the body. Dry fasting is not for everyone, and it isn't easy to do. People can do prolonged extended water fasting, but dry fasting can be done only safely in shorter intervals. I will not recommend for anyone to do it for over eight days. In fact, I would advise people with caution to do one day at a time with a maximum timeframe of three days. Dry fasting in the U.S. and Western countries is not as popular; however, in places like Russia they have clinics where, for health reasons, they supervise dry fasting for up to 10 days. They cure many diseases through dry fasting, but it can be risky and even fatal without supervision.

Pros: Dry fasting burns a lot more toxins and karma in a shorter amount of time. One day of dry fasting equals two days of water fasting.
Cons: Because dry fasting is a lot more intense, you cannot dry fast for

extended periods.

Fruit Fasting

If people have pain in their joints or hands and become fruitarians for a while, it will help them. It is difficult to eat only fruit, but fruit fasting has proven to remove the body's inflammation, thus reducing the pain from arthritis and other diseases. Fruit fasting also helps protect healthy cells and regenerates cells in the body as it nourishes the body through all the nutrients and enzymes from the fruits. Many yogis do fruit fasting, and fruitarians become healthier individuals on earth. Why? Fruits have a lot of sugar, but it is natural sugar. Fruits carry a lot of enzymes because we do not cook the fruits. All the enzymes and vitamins remain in the fruit. Cooking with high heat or overcooking foods kills a lot of enzymes. And when there are fewer enzymes and nutrients in the food, they do not help us much. When you cook, I recommend slow cooking on a low flame; this way, you will keep more enzymes to regenerate your cells.

Fruit fasting is not for everyone, but those with health problems can try it. Try it, and it might work for you. People in India fruit fast for 9-10 days, and they do it twice a year. Until people try it and go through the experience themselves, they will not know what benefit they can get from it.

Even if it is a partial fast, such as eating fruits only, it can be very beneficial. Drinking juices only can create a lot of acid, but fruits have fiber in it, and it cleans your intestines, organs, tissues, and regenerates your cells. I've seen people stay on fruit for maybe one, two, or three years, and not only do their cells regenerate, but their DNA changes too. It is like bleaching the DNA - your blood. The more enzymes and natural things you consume, the more they modify your DNA in a good way. That is why I suggest that people not eat junk food. Sometimes it is okay, but because it has many preservatives and fast food is overheated, there is no nutrition at all. It may taste good, but there are no enzymes. Fruit fasting is a great diet. As yogis, we used to do four to five years on fruit only, so our bodies were very healthy.

When you eat fruits, know not all fruits mix well together. Different fruits digest at various rates, and certain combinations can hinder digestion and create fermentation, toxicity, acidosis, nausea, and headaches. Fruits are typically divided into 4 categories: acid, sub-acid, sweet, and melons. Fruits in the acid category should never be mixed with fruits in the sweet category, and melons should always be eaten alone because of their water content. In general, it is best to eat fruits alone and not mix them with any other food group. Although some fruits like melons digest in ten minutes, some can take up to one hour to digest. That's why it is best to allow one hour to digest fruits. Then you can switch to eating something from another food category. This understanding will drastically improve your digestion and health.

Pros: When you fruit fast, you eat all the fiber from the fruits, which helps digest the fruits better. When you juice the fruit, it loses this benefit. Fruit fasting regenerates the cells and nourishes the body.

Cons: People with blood sugar problems have to be careful. You must clean all fruits thoroughly to avoid ingesting harmful bacteria and pesticides. Also know certain fruit combinations can hurt your system.

Intermittent Fasting

The name "intermittent fasting" is so popular these days. However, partial fasting has been around since the beginning of time. We call it Ekasana or Beasana, you eat one or two meals respectively in one day. The rest of the day, you drink only water. No milk, juice, snacks, or anything else. Just purified water. The current trend with intermittent fasting is fasting for 16 hours and eating for the remaining 8 hours. For example, eating from 12:00 pm - 8:00 pm, and fasting for the rest of the time.

Intermittent fasting has many proven health benefits backed by science, but the body doesn't enter a full rest and cleansing state because you are still consuming heavy foods. You are just giving the body extra time to digest all the food, so it becomes a partial rest and cleanse. It can still give a lot of benefits, like weight loss. Intermittent fasting would be more effective, though, if you also reduced the amount of food you consume and avoid eating heavily toxic foods such as meats, especially pork, beef, eggs, or processed foods. Always eat less than your hunger and don't fill up your stomach too much. These lighter fasts have many health benefits and will keep your body very healthy.

Pros: It gives more time for digestion and helps to burn fat.

Cons: Overeating during eating hours can create digestive problems.

Raw Vegan Fasting

Most raw fruits are okay to be eaten raw, but not all vegetables. Many people eat kale, lettuce, or raw spinach in salads, but something people don't realize or consider is that they can carry harmful bacteria such as E. Coli. Some strains of this bacteria can create potential health risks that can damage your system, which can be very dangerous. In India, leaves or these kinds of vegetables are always cooked or boiled; this way, the bacteria can be killed and not hurt you. It is an excellent system to follow. They never eat raw spinach because they know they can get sick from it. If you eat leafy green vegetables, be sure to wash them individually -- all leaves thoroughly. Even if the package suggests they have been washed, these bacteria can still hide, and you will not see them. This is why greens like spinach and kale are best if you boil or steam them. Raw spinach and other vegetables have concentrated amounts of oxalate, which has been linked to kidney stones formation. Raw vegan diets are a bit too extreme, and instead of benefitting from them, people are getting sick because they do not realize that not all vegetables and certain fruits can be eaten raw.

Generally, you eat fruits raw. But there are certain fruits you cannot eat untreated. Some may have to be cleaned, steamed, or even marinated with lime juice, salt, or chili powder to avoid catching harmful bacteria. Raw vegan can be a good diet, only if people become knowledgeable about these things. Once the person tries it, they will know if it is a suitable type of fast for them or not. If their bodies do not respond well to this diet, they will know because they will have digestive issues. For health reasons, if you wish to follow this diet, you can try it for one month and extend from there only if your body can take it. Also, if your body has too much acid, you must be careful not to eat too many acidic fruits. If people don't have this knowledge and they keep eating it, it will create an imbalance. It is a blessing these days we have the internet to check if what we are eating is acidic or alkaline. If alkaline, it will balance your pH levels. This kind of partial fast can be beneficial when knowledgeable about the risks of eating raw fruits and vegetables and the proper combination of fruits and vegetables.

Another factor to consider when eating raw is learning of the rate at which vegetables and fruits digest. It is not a good idea to eat fruits and vegetables together, and as mentioned, don't mix acid fruits with sweet fruits, and eat melons alone. Allow your body to digest what you are eating properly and according to their digestion rate. Otherwise, you will experience a lot of bloating, gas, nausea, feeling sick, and headaches.

Pros: Partial fasting eating raw vegetables and fruits can regenerate cells.
Cons: Not cooking vegetables or washing them properly can bring harmful bacteria into the body presenting potential health risks. Eating the wrong combinations of fruits and vegetables can create digestive issues.

No Animal Products Fasting

There is a lot of emphasis on becoming vegan or plant-based, which is not to consume or put any animal products and byproducts in the body. Many people don't realize that animals eat dirty grass and drink dirty water, so even if the animal's system digests it, it stays in the meat. If people eat this meat or drink the milk without little processing, they can get sick. It is not so common in India to give cows hormones, but they still boil the milk and use it as soon as possible to avoid it from going rancid. This way, it is less harmful. Boiling it kills all the bacteria.

When people eat a meat-based diet and change to a vegan diet, they immediately get affected. Their health improves drastically. According to *Ayurveda*, a holistic healing system, there are three body constitutions: *Kapha, Pitta, and Vata*, which I will go into more detail in a future chapter. When Kapha is someone's central element, they are not supposed to eat any dairy products. Kapha in Sanskrit means "that which holds things together." When there is too much Kapha in the body, the person quickly gains weight. Kapha can ruin their body and the time will come when anything they eat makes them gain weight, even beans, rice, and grains. Naturally, when a person whose main element is Kapha stops consuming dairy products, they will see a significant change in their weight. Why? Because they stop consuming the fat in the milk. And when it stops, they lose weight.

In Western countries and increasingly worldwide, farmers give bioengineered growth hormones to animals and cows to increase milk production. Those hormones come into the human body through the meat and milk people have. With this kind of milk, notice how children grow suddenly too much. If parents are not even 5 feet tall, kids become 6 feet because of the milk's hormones. In some households, children drink milk like water. Organic milk still has natural hormones, but regular milk has an increased level that will make children develop quickly and mature at an early age.

Before, when there were no such hormones in the body, there was no desire to have sex at a young age. But nowadays, children mature early. Sometimes, even at age 11, they get involved sexually and create babies. It means hormones made them mature enough to feel a sexual desire. This sex desire comes through hormones. I suggest to people, especially in Western countries, not to give your children that kind of milk. If you consume milk, buy organic, certified milk, especially if you have children. When you stop drinking cow milk and switch to vegan milk, you do not have to worry about this at all.

Another side benefit of eating plant-based is that muscles and cells will regenerate. Any time a meat-eater changes to vegetarianism, they will get affected positively. And if vegetarians go into veganism, it will do the same thing. If they cannot lose weight as vegetarians, as vegans they will lose weight. Or, suppose they go from vegetarian to fruitarian. In that case, it will regenerate even more cells. Their body will become very healthy, and that's what I said, even arthritis, or similar kinds of diseases, disappear.

Pros: A vegan fast can help divert inflammation and diseases like cancer, diabetes, heart disease, dementia, and arthritis.
Cons: It will take time for the body to adjust. You might experience gas and feel bloated eating grains, beans, rice, and nuts, but it will pass after some time. Be patient.

Traditional Fasting

There are many ancient traditional fasts. In chapter five, I will give you a specific list of practical fasts you can follow. You will see there are many options to choose from according to what your body can do. Any time there is eating involved, you want to eat light vegetarian foods. If you eat meat or take bone broth, it will be counterproductive to the purification of your soul. Remember, you can start with the simple fasts and slowly progress to more difficult fasts to burn more karma.

Who should fast?

Almost everyone can fast according to their body's condition and ability. Fasting needs to be done in moderation or by merely adjusting certain aspects of food and fluid consumption. For fasting to be effective at the karmic level, you need to be wholly into it. You cannot just fast because everyone is doing it. Fasting by imitation does not burn as much karma. You have to immerse yourself into the fast and flow with it. In addition, your intention for fasting also plays a significant role. I suggest that everyone fasts at whatever degree or level they can according to their body's ability.

For spiritual reasons

If anyone is seeking to uplift their soul and wishing to burn their karma, they should fast. Many sages, ascetics, saints, and spiritual practitioners from the past have fasted significantly. It doesn't matter who we are talking about, Tirthankara Mahavira, Buddha, Jesus, Tirthankara Adinath, Tirthankara Parshvanath, or whoever is on the spiritual path. They all fasted. This list doesn't include people considered the reincarnation of Vishnu or Shiva. People make up stories that Vishnu is like a god. However, he's more like an angel, a *deva*. And Shiva is a great angel, a *maha deva*. So, the people considered incarnations of Vishnu, Rama, Krishna, etc., were not seen fasting.

But people genuinely trying to figure themselves, trying to discover who they really are, always fast. They want to burn their karma to set their souls free. Karma doesn't let us see the reality or truth. Therefore, we need to remove these blockages, curtains, or darkness. This way, all illusion and ignorance can go away to bring clarity. Those who wish to gain clarity by removing these clouds of delusion, ignorance, and darkness should fast.

For health reasons

Anyone carrying this human, physical, or gross body should fast at some point in their lives. The physical body contains a lot of sickness and disease. Each of the millions of pores in the body carries almost one and three-quarters of disease, which is almost two types of disease per pore. This disease is hiding underneath, and we don't know when it will come to the surface. While disease remains hidden, everything is okay, but when it comes up to the surface, revealing itself, people suffer a lot. People don't realize that they can burn that disease before it appears. These days we call it DNA. The unique genetic code of each person is there, and everything is buried in it. In addition, scientists have identified that we carry 100 times more DNA from the microbiota living in the human body than our own.

Fortunately, we can purify this DNA. In fact, the original idea of stem cell research was to purify the DNA. If we can purify this gross body before anything happens to it, we can prevent many things. Fasting purifies the DNA and everyone should experience fasting to some degree, even if it is not a full fast. There are options for everyone; they can eat once per day, drop a meal, juice fast, or have only fruits like Hindus during Navaratri.

Disease and sickness are dormant in the body, so it is best to fast before they surface. The body also needs to rest occasionally. As I have mentioned before, the body is like a machine, and like all machines, the body needs rest. And fasting means rest. In that aspect, I suggest that everyone experiences fasting to prevent sickness and disease. When you fast, you will discover that fasting makes your physical body healthy and happy.

For health reasons, people with addictions should also fast, and almost everyone is addicted to something. I can tell you, though, the biggest addiction in the world is food. Those who fast and stay without food help their physical body and automatically attain willpower. Once people build strong willpower, they can fight and overcome any other addiction. Those with heavy addictions need to fast longer, not just one day. I suggest they try four to eight days. In this sense, even if people do not want to experience the spiritual benefits of fasting, they can at least experience this to eliminate their addictions. Fasting from food helps create the willpower to overcome and break other addictions.

Who should not fast?

Everyone, in general, can try partial fasting but not extended fasting. I consider extended or prolonged fasting abstaining from all food and or water for over 24 hours. For some, even a few hours of fasting can be too much. Those who cannot do extended fasting can always do a few hours daily or reduce food intake and still experience many benefits.

I do not recommend people to do prolonged fasting if they are experiencing any of the following:

- Diabetes
- Advanced sickness or disease
- High blood pressure
- Heart disease
- Pregnancy
- Nursing a baby
- Malnutrition, eating disorders, underweight, anemia

- Extreme acidity, phlegm, or gastric trouble
- Weak immune system
- A non-supportive environment
- Taking medications

What are some reasons why this select group cannot fast?

Diabetes: People with diabetes risk their health when fasting because sugar levels in the blood can fluctuate too much, which can be a severe danger. I suggest for them to do partial fasting only.

High Blood Pressure: People with high blood pressure, when fasting, can disturb their heart. If they fast, they are taking this risk. They can try fasting for a maximum of one day, but I would not suggest longer. Instead, I recommend that they practice partial fasting.

Cancer: During the early stages of cancer, fasting can be tremendously beneficial. There is a big possibility to heal stage I and II cancer. If individuals with cancer juice fast with freshly made juices containing certain herbs, vegetables, and fruits, they can reap many benefits. They can make juices using ginger, lauki (Indian zucchini), berries, celery, and more. It will help nourish the cells where the cancer is growing. Instead of damaging the muscles, flesh, or tissues, these cancerous cells will feed on the juices and renew. People with stage I and II cancer can try to dry fast here and there. This might help to repair the cancerous cells altogether. Fasting repairs old or damaged cells, and stem cells regenerate, producing new and healthy cells in the body. This process can only happen in the early stages of cancer when the body is still strong and not too much damage has been done. It will not be easy and those who try it will have a very difficult time. Doctors may oppose it, but there is a possibility that they can heal themselves. Doctors will say you need medication or chemotherapy, and yes, some people must go through medicines and chemotherapy, but it all depends on the cancer stage.

In higher stages, the cancer is out of control, and fasting is not advisable. In these cases, I do recommend surgery or treatment. Still, you never know, there are some exceptional cases where fasting can cure even stage IV cancer when combined with our special Purnam Yoga techniques. Purnam Yoga is a system I created based on intensive breathing techniques that creates a fire in the body to burn toxins rapidly. Even those with stage IV cancer can do it, and it can help improve their health, and in those exceptional cases, it can even remove cancer. There are no guarantees in life; however, there is a stronger chance of healing fully in the first two stages.

Excessive Acidity: When people have excessive acidity, mucus, or gastric trouble, it is not recommended to do extended or prolonged fasting. These symptoms show there is an imbalance in the body.

When the body contains too much acid it is called acidosis. A healthy pH level of the blood is considered 7.4, and according to the American Association for Clinical Chemistry acidosis happens with a pH of 7.35 or lower. Those with too much acidity in their bodies are not supposed to do prolonged fasting. Even one or two days of water fasting can create trouble for them. As soon as they fast, they experience nausea and vomiting because they have too much acid in their body, and that acid needs to come out. Instead of fasting, there are other natural ways to remove or balance this acidity. In the yoga system, we have special yogic kriyas for that.

As long as this high acidity level remains in the body, I do not recommend fasting. If uncertain about this, you can ask your physician to order blood work for you to determine your blood's pH level, but you need to be clear from it to go into an extended fast. Anyone can tolerate one or two days, but people with too much acidity in their body run a risk of losing their body if they force it longer.

Excessive Mucus: People with abnormal mucus, phlegm, or congestion in their bodies also have a lot of trouble while fasting for extended periods. If they do, it will not be easy, but with strong willpower they can eventually burn the mucus in their bodies. However, this can be quite risky, and those with this condition run the possibility of losing their lives too. And it happens in India. They go into a fast, and they don't listen. They think, "Oh, I can do eight days," and within eight days, they die. Underlying medical conditions can be the cause of having abnormal levels of mucus. I suggest checking your body first. Visit your doctor to find out if it is too acidic or has too much mucus. I do not advise you to enter a long fast until it is clear.

Excessive Gas: The third imbalance is excessive gas or gastric trouble. This imbalance could represent an underlying health problem affecting your digestive system. The gas usually stays trapped in the stomach, intestines, and ribs, and if people with this issue fast for too long, the gas travels to the head, making them mentally unstable. If the body's elements are normal and balanced, then people can go into an extended fast. If not leveled, everyone can try at least one day.

Pregnancy & Nursing: Pregnant women or nursing moms should not fast because they have to think about their baby's needs. The baby needs food. If the mom experiences some sickness, they can change their diet to a lighter diet or do a partial fast. A partial fast can be dropping one meal and drinking water throughout the day, but not a full fast. If pregnant up to two months, they can fast for a maximum of one day, but I don't suggest it after two months because they are hurting the soul growing inside them. Nursing women should not fast because fasting can affect their milk production. Again, partial fasting would not affect much, but extended fasting is certainly not recommended.

Non-Supportive Environments: It is already hard enough to fast, but when you are surrounded by very negative people that do not support your idea of fasting, it can become very challenging. If you are in this situation, it is better not to fast. Avoid fasting in a non-supportive environment and instead fast alone or go to a retreat to have more encouragement, positivity, and support. This is one reason many people visit us at Siddhayatan Tirth & Spiritual Retreat because they want to be in a positive and spiritual environment that encourages and supports their fasting efforts.

Taking Medication: In general, it is never a good idea to fast while taking medications. People taking any drugs to treat psychiatric conditions, diabetes, cancer, heart disease, low sugar, kidney problems, or other grave conditions should not fast, except for short periods at a time or by skipping a meal per day.

Weak Immune System: Anyone with a weak or compromised immune system should not fast. It is not recommended to fast for people with very weak immune systems due to chronic or long-term illnesses. This includes cancer, Hepatitis C, HIV, or auto-immune type of diseases. If the disease has spread too much and death appears to be imminent, fasting can be a last resort for healing. In exceptional and rare cases, it can have favorable outcomes. For example, if the doctor says someone has four months left to live, they have limited time, but they might survive a little longer if they fast.

Can someone with a very toxic body fast for an extended period?

If a person is highly toxic from drinking too much alcohol, smoking, doing drugs, or following a poor diet, I suggest not cleaning their body through fasting *at first*. It is not safe. The first step to detox is to stop taking new toxins in. Changing bad habits and diet will help you next. When you follow an organic vegetarian or vegan diet it will help your liver, kidneys, and digestive system to detoxify your body.

Next, going through an alternative cleansing approach is the best. You can start by doing an enema. It needs to be safely administered or by following a medical professional's instructions. Then follow an herbal and natural system like Ayurveda or Traditional Chinese Medicine. They both focus on health and wellness and offer different methods to heal and cleanse the body. Some treatments include boiling different herbs, which are useful to detox and strengthen the organs and muscles. In Ayurveda, we call this process *kadha*; you boil herbs and spices until you extract all their essence and benefits. About 50% of the water evaporates, and the remains are very powerful, like medicine. That is how Ayurveda cleans the toxins or impurities accumulated in the body.

The next step of the process is to come to the yogic system. In the yogic system, we have something called an "inner bath." An outer bath is easy to take; you go into the shower and clean your body. But an inner bath is very difficult to do. An internal bath is done through kriyas as taught in the yogic system. Soon, I will teach these kriyas at Siddhayatan Tirth to help people cleanse their bodies. We have one kriya called *Kunjal Kriya*. The Kunjal Kriya is similar to an elephant drawing water from its trunk and then splashing it out like a shower. Kunjal means "elephant," and Kriya means "like." In this kriya, we put water in the stomach, mix it, and then throw it out. Many people don't believe acidity can be healed, but with kriyas like this one, it is likely to happen if done correctly. Another method is called *Shankh Prakshalan*. Shankh means "conch," and Prakshalan means "to wash completely." It is like the ocean washing a conch. This technique cleanses your entire alimentary canal, from mouth to colon.

Everything with only water and movement. In the future, I will teach step-by-step how to use these techniques to cleanse the body. The organs and muscles will release and drain all toxins by going through this approach. People's bodies will become like a beautiful flower, and once they do, they will be able to fast smoothly, which will help burn an abundance of karma.

Tirthankara Mahavira, unfortunately, did not know this irrigation system. Otherwise, he could have burnt karma quickly. During his days, this system was not very popular. I have seen no one more stubborn than Tirthankara Mahavira on the Earth. He was very adamant about not following the yogic system. Tirthankara Parshvanath's teachings were available for him to follow and practice, but he was unwilling to adopt these yogic teachings. In the end, he gave up entirely and adopted the yogic system. He was so stubborn that he finally reached enlightenment after sitting for three days in the cow-milking pose. Determined people like him will die before moving. Most people cannot sit for even one minute, and he did three days in the cow-milking posture. At first, he wanted to achieve enlightenment by fasting only, but fasting works only to a certain degree. You cannot, however, deny that other systems can work too and can boost your efforts.

Remember, I recommend finding alternative methods for cleansing very toxic bodies before doing an extended fast. Enemas and colonics can be done sometimes through the guidance of professionals. Anyone can practice yogic kriyas and it will help them have a much smoother fast, which will allow them to burn a lot more karma.

Is extended fasting better than short fasting?

It depends on the person's body. For certain body types, such as those with a lot of acidity, extended fasting is not for them. If they do an extended fast, they will have a really hard time. When people fast, if they do not vomit after one or two days, it indicates that they have lower acidity levels, so they can continue into extended fasting, maybe for 10-15 days and sometimes up to 30 days or more.

In terms of burning karma, short fasting versus extended fasting makes no difference. Both burn the same amount of karma. In just one or two days, the person with an acidic body will experience really low energy, and the fast will be physically challenging. These are symptoms that karma is coming up on the surface. We call it *Udirana*. Udirana is a process in which you force karma to mature and take its course. When the person's body feels sick in one single fast, it shows how that kind of body brings up karma to the surface. Therefore, the karma takes shape as a result. Udirana means you can invite karma quicker by putting effort by voluntarily fasting.

In India, some people do a fast called *Varshitap*. One day they eat, and the next day they water fast. They alternate back and forth during one year. It seems easy, but initially, it is difficult. After a while, the body adjusts; then, it goes smoothly. Varshitap is very popular in the Samanic tradition, and many people from the different Jain branches do it. A more challenging variation of this fast type is *Belatap*, eating one day and water fasting for two consecutive days, also alternating for one year. These are short fasts over a long period, and they are even more difficult than extended fasting. In extended fasting, suppose a person is fasting for one month; mentally, they know that they will break the fast after one month. But the person doing Varshitap or Belatap is fasting and breaking the fast constantly. This steadfast commitment is an invitation for bad karma to give you a result immediately. Hence, making this short fasting a lot more efficient at burning karma than extended fasting.

Does that make short fasting better than extended fasting? By principle, extended fasting is more beneficial, but only when it is safe to do so. However, some people might fast for eight days and achieve the result of someone else doing 30 days. Some people's bodies might not allow them to go beyond eight days, and if they do, they could lose their lives. Many factors affect the result of each fast. All fasts are beneficial, even fasting for two or three days out of the year. But if you can do more, you can achieve more benefits. All fasting burns karma, and soon I will share with you how much karma you burn with even one fast.

Why is it better to heal the body first in order to fast?

Some may wonder, if a person who fasts for one day and can invite many karmas through the suffering they experience, then why fix their body if they already can bring so much karma to the surface? Isn't the fast supposed to heal the body? If a person's body is healthy, they can do more tapa or fasting. If a body is already sick and cannot take too much fasting, it cannot do long-term fasting. Many people cannot even take two days, but they can fast a little longer or go into a longer-term fast if they can tolerate more.

In extended fasting, people also experience pain and other discomforts, but they are not as strong. A person who struggles with a one-day fast cannot do Varshitap fasting. This type of body, which always experiences pain and suffering when fasting, is considered a weak body. It is a weaker body, but it burns a lot more karma than others. However, this type of body cannot tolerate too much tapa. A healthy body can do a lot more tapa, which is why I suggest healing the body first. When you do extended fasting, you can burn a lot of karma too. The body may cooperate, but that doesn't mean the fast is always smooth. Negativities also surface – internal and external. Some people cannot sleep at night, others experience many emotions, and others go through negativities such as anger or hatred. They invite karma in a different way.

In short fasting, they may quickly experience physical pain, but anger and negativities will not be too strong. In prolonged fasting, you stretch the possibility of bringing up deeper negativities to dissolve them. A person could be calm and peaceful when suddenly they blow up while fasting. When emotions and negativities surface, it means the karma is giving you a result, it means the fast is working, and most important, it means it is burning and clearing it from your soul.

What are other benefits for extended fasting vs. short fasting?

There is always a physical benefit when doing short or extended fasting. I can tell you, though, what is not a benefit. Any time you force long fasting when the body cannot take it, it can be dangerous. When you go beyond your body's ability, the muscles become very weak, and the system shuts off, so it is imperative to break the fast before risking your system not waking up. Sometimes people become too stubborn; they get stuck thinking they want to fast for 30 days, but after 20 days, their body is different, and no matter what they do to fix it or push through, they die.

In India, I have seen this happen, even within eight days or less. They force themselves, and they die. They could have done many meaningful things with their lives, but now their body is gone. So, in these cases, extended fasting was not beneficial. People are stubborn. All the signs are there. Their body is uneasy and not cooperative, so it indicates they should not go further. For most people who fast, their idea is only physical health. Physical health is a side benefit. It happens, but if they force themselves too much, it can go the other way around, and they never regain their strength. Once you fast, if you feel uneasy to where you notice your body is not functioning well, you need to break the fast immediately. I strongly suggest not to force fasting. Go according to your body. Listen to it. Be non-violent to it. You always save your body first.

Remember, the longer you have a body, the longer you can burn karma. Your body is your instrument to burn karma, and if you lose your instrument, that's it. Your life is wasted. I am pro-saving your body first. This is why I suggest to everyone to fast one or two days at a time. You will still burn karma and experience many other benefits. When you break the fast, suddenly clarity comes, and clarity is the most significant benefit of fasting. People seeking clarity need to fast according to their body. If their body is healthy and strong, it will help them go further and clarity will come.

Does fasting help create balance on the planet?

Many people, including experts, believe that global warming results from carbon dioxide, pollutants, and greenhouse gas emissions. However, they don't realize that humans contribute to the globe's rising temperatures differently. The land, oceans, and atmosphere are warmer than ever. But is it solely due to external pollutants? No. Sometimes I say that the most significant pollution in the world is our thoughts. And when negative thoughts enter the atmosphere, they directly fuel global warming. Most people in the world have negative thoughts, and according to researcher Dr. Fred Luskin of Stanford University, each human has up to 60,000 thoughts in one day, with 90% being repetitive. As a conservative estimate, at least 80% of people's thoughts are negative. We are talking about almost eight billion people. So, can you imagine how much negativity enters the atmosphere each day? I can guarantee you that if only animals lived on Earth, there would be no global warming. Not only because of the lack of contamination but because animals do not have negative thoughts.

If global warming creates a significant imbalance on Earth, it can have catastrophic consequences. But suppose 100,000 people collectively fast for eight days straight, and they are in a spiritual environment, good mood, positive thoughts, and immersed in spiritual learning and growth. They have no expectations and want to explore themselves spiritually. Automatically, they create positive energy on Earth, and positive energy lacks force and strength. So, imagine what would happen if one million people or more did it together. If they increase positive energy, it will create more balance on the planet. But if no one cares to create positive energy, then the planet will be imbalanced all the time.

The question is, how many people are in the spirit to do it? For example, people sometimes pray at church, maybe a group of 50 to 100. But this is not enough. If we had a fixed time where everyone does prayer, meditation, fasting, or silence simultaneously, this collective effort could create positive energy. Why? Because those doing it are in a positive mindset, higher consciousness, and higher thinking. But what do most people do? They do these things individually. It still helps, but it only contributes on a small scale. However, to have a major and quicker effect on the planet it has to be done collectively.

During Paryushan, a Jain celebration for soul upliftment, people fast collectively. There are 18 days when people engage fully in fasting and spiritual learning, and it creates the highest energy. Soon after, Hindus celebrate the spiritual festival of Navaratri over a 9-night period. They have positive attitudes and are in positive thoughts.

They fast by only eating the lightest and simplest foods like vegetables, fruits, and juices. Even though it is a partial fast, their mood and ambiance are very beautiful. *Dussehra* follows Navaratri on the 10th day, which marks the end of the celebration. Combined, over one billion people partake in that mood, so they automatically create balance for the planet. The same thing happens when Muslims participate in Ramadan. Even though they only stay without food and water during the daytime, they intend to engage in positive thinking and prayer, which also helps create balance.

If anyone truly wishes to contribute to the Earth's overall balance, you can follow the Jain schedule. Millions of people fast during Paryushan. They not only fast, but they also do a lot of meditation, *samayik* (state of being), *pratrikraman* (confession and self-analysis), stay in monasteries, and listen to spiritual lectures from the nuns and monks. Jains who opt to still eat during Paryushan will not eat vegetables because they don't want to harm the vegetation, so they follow non-violence to the best of their abilities. They are in a beautiful mood, and this creates the perfect atmosphere to create positive energy.

It is best to be a part of a collective effort to create more balance on Earth. You can fast during Paryushan or Navaratri. It doesn't matter where your location is. You can do it from anywhere in the world and support this energy. Most important, be in higher thinking when you fast. Don't fight, pray, meditate, read spiritual books, do sadhana, clean your home, wear clean clothes, and altogether it will help.

CHAPTER 5

PERSONAL EXPERIENCE

My experience with fasting begins many lives ago when I was a yogi in the Himalayas. The Himalayas are a fantastic chain of hills with many healing attributes. One day, we were digging the ground and found a special root not connected to a tree. We cleaned the root, cut it, and then ate it. We soon realized this root could remove our hunger for ten days. It was an incredible discovery. After eating it, I could dry fast for ten days continuously. For ten days, there was no need to urinate, go to the bathroom, or anything. This discovery allowed me to sit in a meditative state for ten days straight.

It was challenging to find this root because it was buried underground, and it was not visible. As yogis, we knew how to search for it; however, we were not always lucky. Occasionally, we would find a more potent root, and I could dry fast for up to 21 days. No food and no water. Eventually, we would eat the root and fast for a four to five-month period. These fasts were very difficult to do, but the root would allow us to sustain our bodies and energy for long periods of time without eating or drinking anything.

Tirthankara Adinath, the first Tirthankara, used to reside in the Himalayas. He used to go to Mount Kailash and Ashtapad, the twin hills. In the summer, he would go to Mount Kailash and sit at an elevation of almost 22,000 feet high. In the winter, he would go down to Ashtapad because it was a bit more sheltered. He and his followers must have known about these roots because they would last an entire year with no food and water. They would eat these roots and fast continuously for one year. We would do the same and fast for months. The remarkable root would burn all the toxins in our body, and when there are fewer toxins, fasting becomes effortless.

Toxins make fasting very difficult. This is why I always tell people to clean their bodies before they fast. Even though the fast removes toxins, if the body is full of heavy toxins, it can create a lot of trouble when you start fasting, especially if you are doing an extended fast. For long-term fasting, it is best to prepare yourself as we did for ten days. Because the heavy toxins burn, you will be astonished at how smoother your fast goes. Your body becomes like a flower, and you can survive for one or two months with water only—nothing else.

What would you do while fasting?

We lived in the Himalayas, and I would do a lot of spiritual practices, meditate, walk around, and enjoy nature. Nothing bothered us. We lived in so much peace, and there were no outside people or distractions. It was all simple and beautiful. It was complete nature. Sometimes we would go to the caves for shelter or sit under the trees. While fasting, though, I would experience a lot of pain as I invited my karmas to come up. In the earlier days of fasting, I would go through many difficulties because I didn't have the right knowledge about fasting. I would not clear my stomach before fasting, which would create a lot of trouble for me. Because of these terrible experiences, I strongly suggest that you empty your stomach first, this way you don't have to go through what I went through.

How did you transition into your current body?

During my last life as a yogi, I had the current weak human structure called *asamprapta strupatica sanhanana*. Within the human instrument, there are stronger and weaker bodies, as I mentioned before. As a yogi in the Himalayas, we used to travel a lot -- astral travel, also known as out-of-body experiences. One day, during my astral travel journeys, I went too far. Perhaps, many galaxies away from where my body was located. Unfortunately, my body became damaged in my absence and I had little time remaining. Because of the lack of time and because I still had *Ayu Karma* (lifespan karma) remaining, I was left with two choices. One choice was to enter moksha or liberation through a painful technique and the other option was to enter another body.

Luckily, as a yogi, I knew how to enter someone else's body. However, two main souls cannot stay in one body. Occupying another body only works if one soul is exiting and one is entering. I had only one hour to find a body to enter into, and it needed to be a pure body. Fortunately, I found one. Simultaneously, a young Jain monk was dying, and everyone had lost hope he would survive. The monk's soul was departing his body, and I began the process to enter his body. I chose his body because he had never even tasted meat, eggs, or anything bad. It was what I was looking for because yogis are very particular. Real yogis will never suggest to anyone eating meat products because they know it takes years to clean their bodies afterward.

This body was frail when my soul took over it, and I had to do many yogic practices to restore it. It took me approximately six months to heal, invigorate, and strengthen it. It was a sick and ailing body dying due to improperly breaking a 32-day fast. The monk's teacher was not knowledgeable about safely breaking the fast, so the monk did not eat according to his body's condition after such a strenuous and long fast. Had I not been a yogi, I would not have made it into the body I have now. But I made it. I had to do many intense ancient techniques like *Kapalbhati* and *Anulom Vilom,* among other techniques, to heal and strengthen it. Everyone around me thought I was the same person, except for the boy's teacher. He knew I was different. He would say I was not the same and that I knew everything. He would ask, "Is it really you? What happened to you?"

He was doubtful about who I was because I gave lectures differently, and he would ask where I learned those things because he had never taught me that.

Eventually, I had to leave the teacher and go on my own. I continued my journey as a Jain monk, teaching the Jain system and the yogic system. I combined both because the Samanic tradition is also part of the yogic system, so I knew both systems.

Can you recollect your current body's experience with fasting?

My experience in the Himalayas was different from what my current body endured through the 32-day fast. When one goes through the rare process such as the one I described, they can still connect and speak to the experiences and memories of the body they now live in, and my experience in this body with extended fasting was one with many challenges.

As a young monk, I wanted to experiment with fasting and learn more about myself in a special way. I didn't really want to fast. However, I wondered how long could I survive without food. I was only 14 years old, and I thought the maximum I could survive was eight days, and the next thing I knew, I was taking a vow not to break my fast until the eighth day. I was determined that I would finish no matter what. I did not know what to expect and was unaware that things would turn for the worse. The first day went well, but day by day, pain took over my body. After the fourth day, I had severe pain from head to toes. Persistence kept me going as I felt I could reach day eight. Besides, I didn't want to break my vow. Suddenly on the seventh day, I woke up, and my body felt like a flower. The pain had vanished completely. The real fast, for me, began on that seventh day. The fast may start on the fourth, fifth, or maximum, the sixth day for other people. But I had to go through so much more to reach that point. I had a lot of patience and didn't give up. By this time, my hunger had almost disappeared. And on the eighth day, when it was time to break, it was as if I was not even fasting. So, I thought maybe I could go on for nine days. I extended my vow with my teacher one day at a time. I just kept going.

After two weeks, my fast became very strict. I decided not to shower, clean my teeth, or anything. I let nature take its course and decided not to talk or see anyone. The other monks would knock on my door, leave hot water outside, and I would take it as needed. Around the second week, an idea entered my head. I wondered how yogis can sit under the sun without clothes. And I thought I would try it. After two weeks of fasting, something unique happened. I sat outside under the sun at noon every day. It was the hottest time of the day, and it was happening right in the Indian summer. I would go to the roof and sit in the sun. The bricks on the roof were burning hot, and I would sit in meditation at 100 degrees Fahrenheit.

People from the local town discovered what I was doing, and out of curiosity, they would go to the neighbor's homes to take a peek. It was a medium-sized town in Punjab with a population of maybe 100,000, and many people would come out to see me. What was striking about this experience is that my skin would not burn. Instead, my body took food from the sun directly. I would sit in Lotus pose for one to two hours each day. The days would continue to pass and I just kept extending it. I was full of energy, and I would go back to the sun each day for a few hours. People were always mesmerized by how yogis would sit in the sun for hours without burning, and then I realized that the body sucks the energy from the sun. The sun's energy was feeding my body while my hunger and pain evaporated. It was an incredible experience.

I completed 32 days when I broke the fast. After breaking, more amazing things happened. Substances that stay in the stomach while you fast clear after you break it, and once this happens, you feel even better and lighter. It was as if my body had become a baby's body. At age 14, I knew what it felt like to have a baby's body. It was marvelous. Unfortunately, that feeling didn't last too long. Soon after, everything changed. My teacher was not knowledgeable on how to safely refeed my body, so I got very sick. I was not a master then. After two months of breaking the fast, this body began to die. As a yogi, I would know what to do, but the soul in the body didn't. What I truly think happened was that the karmas that surfaced from the young monk's fast attacked right away. That karma was supposed to occur and clear after many births, maybe 500 lives, but they all came up and presented themselves, and as a result, made the body sick.

Understand that breaking the fast is very critical. If you wish to experience having a baby's body and breath, I suggest going into a long fast without forcing it. Attaining a pure body like a baby is possible through fasting. It happened naturally with me. My fast was a strict one because I wanted to go the hard way to experience something more profound. Because I was already a monk, I was used to discipline, but I do not suggest doing it this way these days. It might give you little energy to brush and clean your body. This experience taught me this body is not a body. It is merely an instrument you can use for a higher purpose, for spiritual growth, and that it doesn't require a lot of food.

Why do you continue to fast as a master?

Pollution is in the environment we live in. Even if you are a master, you still inhale and eat contaminants that can affect your body. This is the reason it is essential to fast. No matter who you are, it is beneficial to remove any accumulated toxins from this pollution.

The body comprises bones, tissues, marrow, organs, muscles, and different systems, like the nervous system, and they can all be affected by pollution. If you live in a pollution-free environment, you have fewer chances of getting sick. However, even an enlightened person can get ill and suffer a lot. Why? There is something called *Vedniya Karma*. Vedniya Karma is a feeling-producing type of karma responsible for all the pleasure and pain we feel. There are two kinds of Vedniya Karma: *Shata Vedniya* and *Ashata Vedniya*. Shata means "pleasure or happiness," and Ashata means "pain or misery." And this karma doesn't leave the person until the end of their body. Essentially, it stays with you until the end of your life. Enlightened masters have dissolved their major and heavy karmas, but the lighter ones remain, creating little trouble here and there because of the environment they live in. Enlightened masters like Tirthankara Adinath preferred to be in places like Mt. Kailash or Ashtapad to be in the purest environments. If they stayed in the cities, they would not get affected much because there wasn't much pollution those days, but they would go to the Himalayas if they did get affected. This is how Tirthankara Adinath, with all his 84 chief disciples and students, lived. It was amazing.

Will you leave your body sooner if you fast a lot?

Masters do not leave their bodies sooner if they fast. After enlightenment, you do little fasting, but you do it sometimes to maintain a healthy body for the reasons I've mentioned. I fast during Paryushan and occasionally throughout the year, as needed. The pollution in the environment is not good for you. Enlightened people's age is fixed. They do not get killed by bombs, bullets, crucifixion, serious illness, or accidents. They leave their body differently. So, to know if someone was enlightened in the past, see if they were killed by any of the circumstances I mentioned, then it shows if they were really enlightened or not.

If a spiritual practitioner was killed in the aforementioned ways, it doesn't mean they were not good people or good teachers. They, however, were just not necessarily enlightened. Why? Because enlightened people know what to do if something bad is coming. They will escape those situations and save other people too. It is a different concept. But again, even enlightened masters fast. Tirthankara Mahavira was fasting even after enlightenment, but maybe because he was sitting a lot. If you sit all day, your body doesn't have a lot of movement, so it is better to fast, walk, do yoga, and pranayama to keep your blood circulation and body in good condition. In old age, people lose a little grip on their health, even enlightened masters. Old age is old age, and fasting is always good to maintain good health.

What are the biggest benefits you have experienced while fasting?

The most significant physical benefit I experienced through fasting is my body becoming light like a flower floating. When you fast, you purify your body, dispose of toxins, clear your senses, and remove infection and sickness. It makes your body feel light. Fasting, no matter who you are, takes care of your body. It removes the toxins accumulated from the pollution in the environment and the particles of negative people around you. These particles are floating around you. There are a lot of negativities floating around. People are full of anger particles, and suddenly you can pick them up. And no matter if it is Tirthankara Adinath or Mahavira's time period or these days, bad people are always around. Bad people's negative energy is powerful, and it can affect others.

After fasting, my senses cleared, and they became functional. Once they clear, they have no desires. Your senses become pure like those of babies. And when you are pure, now you can experience the most significant spiritual benefit I experienced, which is to enter the highest states of consciousness in a meditative state. When your senses are clear, and you are a grown-up, that is the time you can actually enter a deep meditative state, and people miss this part. The problem is that if you do not have a teacher to guide you, your experience will be superficial. In Eastern and Western countries, people fast a lot, but they do it for the wrong reasons. They do experience having a light body, but they don't understand that the light body is the only vessel that allows you to enter a full meditative state. So, they miss that phenomenon. Those who receive guidance or have knowledge about it will never miss that experience at all.

Meditation in Sanskrit is *dhyana*. And dhyana is an *agni*, which means fire. If you enter a deep state of meditation, you can burn a lot of your karma in one hour. But this real meditation doesn't happen often. Most people experience superficial meditation. Real meditation only happens when your senses are clear and your body is light—no toxins in the body. The greatest benefit of fasting is achieving the deepest state of your consciousness. If you hit it, you can burn an abundance of karma, which is truly the most beneficial aspect of fasting.

People are satisfied with obtaining a physical benefit from fasting. But those who are knowledgeable about the most significant spiritual benefits are not. They become satisfied only when they can use their light body to enter a deep meditative state. In a deep meditative state, all mysteries unfold. Dark, ignorance, and illusion all disappear. That is why a light body is necessary to enter deep meditation. My experience while fasting was realizing this body is not a body; it is an instrument. You can use it for a higher purpose, and it requires little food. I experienced what Tirthankara Mahavira experienced in his 5-

month-and-27-day-fast. I experienced the same thing in 32 days. This is the real benefit of it. Meditation creates a fire, and once your karma is burnt, everything becomes crystal clear. You see the reality, and you never go backward. You only move forward.

PART II:

SPIRITUALITY

CHAPTER 6

SPIRITUALITY & FASTING

To understand fasting, you must first understand spirituality. Real spirituality is going beyond the experience of life. It is a realization of soul. When you or any person realizes that a soul holds infinite knowledge, that person discovers that substance within them. As they continue on the road of self-discovery, they will be taking steps towards spirituality. All spiritual people are compassionate, loving, evil-less, nonviolent individuals similar to non-extreme religious people, yet they are more refined. Each religion has an aspect of spirituality in it. For example, there are mystics in Hinduism, Islam has Sufism, Christianity has mysticism, and Judaism has Kabbalah. When you refine religion, it becomes spiritual like a fragrance. The fragrance is more valuable than the flower. That fragrance is hidden inside of you. That fragrance needs to be found through *sadhana*.

Sadhana can be a single technique or a variety of techniques that improve your soul every day. It is like your inner flame is expanding every day. Your soul is awakening every day. The more spiritual a person becomes, the more awakening happens from moment to moment. Spirituality means total transformation. The person is not the same anymore. It transforms their energy and transforms their way of thinking. In doing so, they totally change. Their look is different. It is a physical, mental, and spiritual transformation.

The children of our society need this fragrance of spirituality. Society will be different if we become spiritual. Fighting and wars cannot happen where there is spirituality. There is no division. Spirituality is beyond color, race, creed, gender, orientation, religion, etc. The taste of spirituality is the same, whether you are African, Hispanic, Asian, or European. It is like blood. Spirituality is like blood. Blood is red no matter what color skin you have. It is like water. Whoever drinks the water quenches their thirst. Whoever tastes spirituality will light themselves. You cannot treat spirituality like a crutch. You have to be independent. You have to be your own lamp to awaken yourself, to awaken society. That is 100% true. Once you are awakened, you will awaken many people.

Spirituality begins with you. When your soul begins to wake up, your spirituality begins. Curiosity about discovering who you are can make you a spiritual person if you find the right guidance. If your parents are religious, they will only make you religious, and religion is hard to break away from. You can be spiritual if a teacher can hit you at the core of your being and guide you. Even a few words from them can create chaos inside you and cause your being to want to wake up. You think, "Who am I? Where did I come from? Where will I go after I die?" This curiosity can create chaos inside you. When your being wakes up, you know yourself, and all the misconceptions will be dissolved. You will ask, "What is the power working beyond my senses? Was my imagination present before I was born?" When you work with yourself, you will know that you were not born with the mind or the thinking. You were born pure because your soul is pure. To go towards that purity, you have to go step by step.

Soul is like a mirror that shows no reflection when someone steps in front of it. There is no karma, no mind, and no imagination, not even bliss. It is pure. When you say bliss, it means no bliss exists; therefore, it is still in duality. The mind is like a junkyard. We keep filling it with information. If we use the mind to understand, then it is a good instrument. But the mind needs to be cleaned up. Once it is purified, there is no reflection in the mirror because there is no object. When there is no object, spirituality begins. All beliefs are like objects. Where there are objects and thinking, there is a reflection in the mirror.

If you can just be, all the thoughts, beliefs, and karmas will leave you. Can you be in that state of consciousness? That state makes you spiritual. You are a blank slate. When you dive deep into your being, you will find purity there. Fasting helps to remove the mirror's reflection, and it makes you light. The lighter you become, the more you can dive deep, and the deeper you go, the more spiritual you become. Be like a mirror without reflection, with no object, and you are already spiritual.

How does non-violence relate to spirituality?

The first step of spirituality is non-violence. First, you must learn to practice non-violence in your life. Non-violence *(ahimsa)* is when you are in oneness with all living beings. View the world as your family. If you know that all livings beings are your family, you would not hurt or kill them.

The first step of non-violence is to be vegetarian. Being vegetarian is a requirement for total liberation. Eat fruits, vegetables, grains, and beans. Mother Earth provides so much vegetation, and there is no need to kill animals to fill your stomach. Killing animals is a form of violence and accumulates a lot of karma. When you eat meat, poultry, and seafood, you support the industry, perpetuating the supply and demand cycle, causing more deaths to animals, and collecting more karma to block your soul.

Vegetarianism is the first step towards spirituality because it allows one to respect all living beings. To kill animals for food causes them a lot of pain because animals have senses and minds. The killing stresses their whole system, creating adverse reactions, like the release of adrenaline in their blood. This is torture. The person eating the meat of the animal killed will receive all these bad feelings. Vegetables are one-sense-beings, considered the lowest category of food. Choose the lowest form of living beings for your survival because they are unconscious. Even then, only eat what you need.

Being a vegetarian and eating only fruits, vegetables, and grains makes digestion easy on the body. Meat takes about three days to pass through the entire digestive system. Light food brings about a light mind, and a light mind helps in meditation to experience states of *samadhi*, the highest states of consciousness.

It is a wrong notion that meat is good for the brain. Many geniuses and important contributors from the past were vegetarian. Albert Einstein, Pythagoras, Susan B. Anthony, Isaac Newton, Rosa Parks, Nikola Tesla, Gandhi, Tirthankara Mahavira, and Buddha were all vegetarian. Vegetarianism means *satvik*, divine. Thoughts are pure, and with spiritual guidance, a person can be very good. Vegetarian food comes directly from the soil. In this way, you have direct contact with the Earth--the mother that provides everything. It means you respect the Earth and you are divine. Your thoughts are focused in the right direction. Practice non-violence by being vegetarian, and not only will you save many lives every year, but you will also not collect karma and bring impurities into your body.

After vegetarianism, you can practice non-violence in your communication, thoughts, and actions. Break your habit of using bad words. They are unnecessary, and they can be hurtful. Watch the words you use. Don't scream or yell. Speak nicely. Be aware of the thoughts you have. Be away from negative thinking or violent thoughts. If you begin to think negatively or violently, change your thinking immediately to something positive or recite divine sounds – also known as *mantras*. Be non-violent in your actions. Be watchful where you are walking. By walking without awareness, you can hurt living beings. Don't crush spiders or ants. Instead, you can put them in a cup and take them outside. It is not their fault they are lost. Put into practice any preventative methods that will keep bugs out of your home. If you leave food out and it attracts ants, you will collect karma for being careless and now having to kill hundreds of ants. Remember, you are ultimately responsible.

In following spirituality and non-violence, if one is truly pursuing *dharma* (the truth) and freedom, there are specific actions and trades that one should refrain from. Avoiding them also prevents your soul from collecting more karma.

Actions

• Violence (hurting, harming, killing any living being)
• Eating meat (pork, beef, poultry, seafood, egg, or any animal)
• Gambling
• Big lies
• Hunting
• Taking what's not yours
• Smoking, drinking alcohol, taking drugs
• Prostitution or pornography (participating, watching, or supporting it)

Trades

• Fermentation – it creates millions of bacteria.
• Sealing wax – it emits toxic vapors and takes away the lives of bees.
• Alcohol – it creates responsibility for someone's life.

• Heat and fire – working with fire all day long is detrimental to one's health and creates pollution.
• Cutting down trees – it destroys the environment.
• Bringing up women, men, animals, or eunuchs as slaves.
• Cutting animal carcasses.
• Skinning animals for the fur trade.
• Trades in bones, ivory, horns, etc.
• Selling birds and animals.

Everything creates some form of violence. However, these acts can significantly, directly or indirectly, hurt you, other living beings, and the environment.

As the 24th Tirthankara Mahavira once said, *"Live and let others live."*

If someone can follow non-violence fully, they can be a step ahead towards liberation. Non-violence is the first step towards liberating your soul. It connects you to others. Even negative thoughts are considered violence. If you harm someone physically, mentally, or by speech, you carry out violence. If you stay away from these, then you are following non-violence.

Awareness is key in this process. If you are walking, talking, eating, or sleeping with awareness, you will not collect karma. If you have awareness, you cannot hurt any living thing because it has a soul. It feels pain; it has a mind and senses, even if they are perhaps not as developed as our own. Instead of giving pain, give compassion and love. This leads you towards becoming a liberated soul, a *Siddha*, your ultimate goal.

How does non-violence relate to fasting?

There is a deeper meaning attached to the concept of fasting. The practice of fasting is tied to non-violence. Sometimes, in India, fasting and non-violence are practiced to such an extreme that even water is not taken during the fasting period to save the life of living organisms present in water. But this is extreme. A few days of dry fasting are good, but it is not good to go that far because it can be dangerous. When you fast, you give the food you don't consume back to nature or other animals and humans. By fasting, you are giving. The greatest notion of non-violence is that we give back the breath of life to others or nature. The greatest act of non-violence is to let other lives go free, to grant them the freedom to live. This notion is called *abaya daan*, which translates to "granting lives the freedom to exist."

A king once appointed his ministers to office and appointed his son as Secretary of State. The son was the brightest of all of the ministers. One day, the king asked them what the cheapest thing in the world was. One minister said that food was the cheapest thing. Another thought about the first minister's answer and decided that food was not the cheapest thing because it takes a farmer a lot of time and effort to produce the food. He said that meat was the cheapest thing because all you had to do was to shoot the animal with a bow and arrow, and the meat would be ready to be eaten. But the son thought about it and said that he needed more time to decide. He told his father he would give his answer the next morning. Word soon spread that the king's son would speak the next day, and many people gathered in anticipation.

The son left that night and went into the woods. Around midnight, he approached the house of the first minister, who saw him coming. The minister opened his door with surprise and asked if he could be of any help. The king's son told the minister that the king had fallen ill, and the only thing that could save his life was two ounces of human meat from the heart. The minister was shocked and said to the son, "I am sorry, but I cannot do that. However, I am a rich man, and you can take all the gold that you want, as long as you don't tell the king what I have done." The son collected all the gold and left. He went to the next minister's house and asked for two ounces of human meat from the heart. The minister responded in the same manner, and the son again left his house with a lot of gold. He continued going to all of the ministers' homes and ended up with a lot more gold. The next morning, all of the people were anxiously waiting for the son's reply. He appeared before the king and told all the gathered people, "I do not think that meat is the cheapest thing in the world. In fact, meat is the most expensive thing I could find." After that, he brought all the carts of gold he had gathered in front of the king. The king was surprised and asked where this gold came from. His son told the whole story in front of all of his ministers.

If we are so protective of ourselves, we ought to respect all other life too. Even the little ant is afraid for its life when you bring your finger next to it. It runs away. All living things have feelings. All life is to be respected. It is necessary to eat, but we can spare animals' lives by not eating meat. Do we thank the tree for the fruit it gives us so freely? We are eager to thank the person who gives us water, but we neglect to thank the trees and vegetation. We have to develop that degree of gratitude, respect, and love.

Fasting directly connects you to non-violence. When you fast, think of the bigger impact you are creating by not engaging in any form of violence. It is a beautiful thing, and it can lift you up in ways you never imagined. Allow your soul to experience this incredible feeling of love, compassion, respect, and oneness.

What is the connection between truth and spirituality?

To know the truth, a true seeker must take a backward journey into the depths of consciousness. Real truth, the real treasure, is hidden there. In this discovery, seekers realize the soul, *atma*. Atma is the consciousness looking, listening, and remembers all things like feelings and memories. Real truth seekers will focus on that substance. The true journey is towards the soul.

Once you become a truth seeker, you will know what to do. You must go on the inward journey. You have to see who you really are. Disconnect all the senses from the outer world. The inner journey is like going backward. You will be going beyond the body, thoughts, and mind. There you will feel something special – maybe your soul, your atma, which knows everything. The soul is beyond body and mind. The real truth seeker becomes peaceful, loving, non-violent, and compassionate.

The soul is the abode of all great qualities. You can feel it. And if you are ever around a highly spiritual person, you will see those qualities in them. The real truth seekers on Earth can be counted. Never become a follower because followers seek outside of themselves. Genuine truth seekers, those who search for their own souls, are very rare. Most people are solely concerned about others. They seek truth in others, but they never seek it within themselves. The day they look at themselves, they have taken a small step towards the truth. The truth seeker seeks within. Truth is within. You are the truth. You exist; you are truth. Find out who you really are.

If one does not know oneself, one commits a crime against oneself. Your life is incomplete if you do not know yourself. Everyone, at some point, asks, "Who am I? How can I know myself?" To know yourself, you need a teacher who will shine a light on your ignorance. They can help light your soul. An enlightened master can provide you with the way to finding the truth. Even though you must walk your own path, the master will guide you like a finger pointing to the moon. Although the moon is visible, that does not mean you can reach it without putting forth effort.

As you search for the truth, I suggest that you consider these questions:

- Who am I?
- Who am I without the things I've acquired?

- Could there be more to this life?
- Could there be more to myself?
- What is real happiness?
- What is real success?
- What is real love and compassion?
- How can I truly become peaceful?
- How do I know myself?

If you know yourself, you are peaceful and satisfied. Try to look at yourself. People want to meet God, but they are trying to know others first. If you meet your soul, you meet God.

What is soul?

The universe is beginningless. The principle of existence proves itself - it was always there. Soul is a power behind energy or matter. When the two come together, they create forms - humans, plants, animals, or nature. There is life everywhere, soul and matter coming together. This is called *jivatma*. Soul minus matter, pure soul, is called *paramatma* or God. God did not create the universe. It existed, it exists, and it will always exist. The laws of physics apply to both soul, energy, and matter alike.

Soul is not a subject that can be researched; it has to be discovered. To come upon this discovery, understand that it is difficult. It takes a lot of effort and energy. The discovery of the soul is like diving into the deep ocean of your consciousness. Most people only sit on the shore; they do not jump in. These people represent the majority of society. They are afraid to discover their true selves, afraid to dive into the unknown. Fearful and weak people are afraid to discover the soul, because it is like death. They fear the end of their previous state of being, of once perceived beliefs and truths. That's why those who try to follow the teachings of enlightened ones, such as Tirthankara Mahavira, discover it.

Atma, or soul, has immense knowledge, great power, and sensation. It experiences pain, suffering, and pleasure. Whatever you think and feel resides in the soul. It originates from the soul. But you can only know the soul, achieve the realization of soul, if you dive deep into your consciousness. That is why I say, "Understand the soul, know the soul, and meditate on soul." Once you know it, you can know yourself. Soul is shapeless and beyond the limitations of words; this is an obstacle for a person. This is the subject of realization. Soul is timeless - it does not move in time or ages. It exists with no beginning.

Soul is the light inside of you. It is the force that drives the body. Even if the organs and senses are still present, the body cannot be alive without this light. Understand that soul, or atma, can be elevated to *mahatma*, the great soul, and to *paramatma*, the expanded soul or consciousness. When you expand your soul, you achieve real peace. When this peace is achieved by following spirituality, you can bring peace to the world. First, be a peaceful person yourself. Don't try to change others; change yourself first.

To work on yourself and raise yourself from jivatma to paramatma,

God, you have to separate matter from soul. You have to destroy your karma. Karma is a subtle matter. By doing sadhana, one day, you will realize that matter and energy have always existed. Soul and matter are eternal - beginningless and endless.

Unfortunately, the soul is surrounded by ignorance, attachment, darkness, and karmas. That is why the discovery of the soul is overwhelming for some. This feeling depends on the senses and the mind. But if soul awakens, if inner awakening happens, then discovery is not far away. It is not even one step away from you. That is why I say you have to take the step towards discovering your soul.

For eternity, the soul has been covered by karma, by darkness. One must remove all of the darkness, all the karma. To do so, one must perform sadhana, or spiritual practices, and tapas - fasting. These techniques will remove all the layers of karma. It is why you want to fast as much as you can in this lifetime for as long as your body allows you to. After this, soul becomes like a free bird. It is free from the traps of karma and darkness. It awakens, and the awakened soul is the real soul.

When you go on the inward journey, you experience many things. This is what Jesus meant when he said, "I am the way." The human body is the door to find yourself. The inner eye is waiting for you. It will open up. The deeper you go inwardly, the more you will find that you are not male or female, white or black, gay or straight. You are the purest soul. You are spiritual.

A person becomes an Arihanta, or enlightened master, when their ego is completely dissolved, totally finished. Arihanta has two words, "ari" which means enemy, and "hanta" which means destroyer. The person who has destroyed all their enemies. The real enemies are the inner enemies: greed, anger, hatred, deceit, jealousy, violence, emotions, and all negativity. They make people's lives miserable. Thus, the person who works on themselves for years or lives, and one day they achieve the highest state of consciousness, becomes an Arihanta. If the mind or senses are present, they do not affect him or her. They are not heavy on his or her soul. The soul, only, is in charge. If a person becomes his or her own master, their soul is awakened and guides the senses, mind, and body. The mind or body does not guide the soul. A master can lift someone else's heart. When this happens, they begin to sprout spiritually.

How does fasting, soul, and spirituality intertwine?

The soul is like a light trapped in karma. Karma is not what we think. It includes many things, such as ignorance, illusion, hallucination, negativities, and blockages. It is like a curtain, hindrance, or cloud that blocks your light. These layers of karma are so thick and dense that they do not let the soul see anything. The more karma we collect, the more karmic particles fuse together. They build on top of each other, creating layers upon layers. With so much density, knots form on top of the layers, and those are very difficult to break. The soul remains in the dark for centuries and centuries, sometimes for hundreds of thousands of years.

You may wonder how to remove these layers and knots. Fasting is one of the best ways to help you achieve this. As soon as people fast voluntarily, if their body allows, they destroy these layers. Layers are easier to remove compared to the knots. Knots are very strong; they are like a nail in the wood. How can you remove a deep nail in the wood? You might have to burn the whole piece of wood, or to remove the nail only, you must put a lot of effort to take it out. If people wish to be in the light and have a lot of clarity, they must burn those knots.

The karmic knots I am referring to are called *granthi*. This is why we call the person on the spiritual path a *Nigrantha*, which means "no knots." Why? Because the knots begin to break. How? They fast. The absolute best reason to fast is to break these karma granthis or knots.

I will explain how this works by giving you an example. Usually, cobra-like snakes love to stay wrapped around the *Chandan* trees, or sandalwood trees. Where there are sandalwood trees, there are always snakes, not only because they like the fragrance, but because they seek coolness, and sandalwood trees are very cool. It is why they wrap their body around the trees to feel the coolness. However, as soon as they see a peacock, their body loosens, and they lose their grip. They fear peacocks, so when they see one, their strong grip becomes weak. They lose their grip, and they don't have time to escape.

Similarly, when you fast, the karmic knots become loose, similar to when the snake's skin becomes loose when they see a peacock. Fasting becomes the peacock, and the granthis become the snake's body. The granthis begin to fall automatically like the snake's body falls from the tree because they are so scared of the peacock. They don't have time to save themselves. In the same way, karma has no time to save itself with fasting. However, it has to be intensive fasting, similar to the fasting Tirthankara Mahavira used to do.

Tirthankara Mahavira's soul had so much dense and intense karma that he did a five-month-and-twenty-seven-day dry fast, and he still could not burn it all. He had so much. Infinite. Forget about us and how much karma we have. Even an extraordinary soul like Tirthankara Mahavira was surrounded by so much karma he had to fast a lot. He did spiritual practices for twelve and a half years continuously, and eventually, he broke all these knots. Once the knots are detangled, the layers peel automatically. But the knots are what keeps the layers together. Once we remove those karma granthis, our soul begins to see through because the layers loosen. The karma is not so intense, so the light passes through.

Suppose there are infinite layers, and out of the infinite, we can loosen up 100,000 layers. The layers are still there, but they are now loosened. That is the time when you get a human body. It doesn't mean you are spiritual yet. But at least you have improved enough to get the best instrument, which is the human body. The human body is considered the best instrument to grow spiritually. At that point, if anyone can receive guidance from someone enlightened or someone else on the right path, slowly, they will improve more and more.

I have known people who fasted once in their life, only one day. And that was all they could do. At least they did something and that is the best thing. I suggest that you try it at least once. If your body doesn't allow it, don't worry. Just break the fast right away. At least you tried. Then try again. And again. When you try and try, eventually, it will happen one day. Don't give up. People who give up are weak people. Always try. It might bring the light right in front of you. Clarity too. You might be able to burn all the acidity in your body. You never know. But I suggest not to force it. If you feel like you are forcing it too much, then only do a little. It is very good to break these karmic knots, they are very strong and stubborn, but brave people can break them.

CHAPTER 7

KARMA & FASTING

If you wish to fast and break the karmic granthis mentioned in the previous chapter, it is essential to precisely understand karma and where these knots come from. Most people are confused about the concept of karma. It doesn't matter if you are from the West, East, or just the general population. Most people lack an understanding of the real karmic theory. Most people are familiar with the notion of good or bad karma, but not the fundamental concept of it.

The real concept of karma is not solely the result of action, mind, or thoughts. To collect karma, first, you need three things: body, mind, and speech. If someone does bad things with their physical body, they collect bad karma, and if someone does good things, they collect good karma. If someone uses abusive language or says something harmful to someone else, they collect bad karma. The opposite can be said for someone who uses sweet and compassionate speech, they will collect good karma. These are the leading causes–body, mind, and speech. However, by these three alone, one cannot collect the profound good or bad karma that can change someone's life.

For karma to have a serious effect on someone, something else is needed. The body, mind, and speech alone cannot bring about any result of grave consequences. A fourth element is required to produce a serious result of karma. That element is intention. This is the aspect that most Western and Eastern thinkers are missing, and intention is the most important aspect of karma. It determines whether the result will have a good or bad effect on someone's life.

If you intend to hurt someone and you enjoy hurting that person, you will collect serious bad karma, and the result will be equally severe. Even if a person intentionally or knowingly thinks about hurting or killing someone, they will collect extremely bad karma, and the result will be the same or similar. If you consciously try to hurt someone with your speech, you will collect a lot of bad karma. But you can say the opposite if you maintain a good body, mind, and speech. If you engage in good actions, thoughts, and speech, you will collect good karma with good intentions. This is the reason intention is very important.

Sometimes people fight to protect someone or themselves, and they may kill someone. The person who was fighting or ended up killing someone does not collect serious karma because, in this case, they intended to defend and not to kill. This is an example of a saying in Sanskrit, *"bhavana bhav naashini,"* if your intention is pure, your birth and life cycle is over. Your suffering has ended. So always remember to keep your intentions pure.

Aside from mind, body, speech, and intention, there is still one more important aspect that can take you to a deep place of suffering: mental activities. If someone is involved in mental activities, day in and day out, planning to hurt or kill someone, or simply thinking negative about others, they will collect immense bad karma for every hour they spend doing so. Activities are more dangerous than your actions, thoughts, and speech. If someone can control their mental activities, especially their destructive activities, they are already safely on the path to awakening. Once you stop or reduce the amount of mental activity, you can stop collecting karma.

We collect many types of karma, but there are eight major karmas. First is that which prevents knowledge, *Jnanavarniya Karma*. The second is that which blocks your right vision, *Darshanavarniya Karma*. The third one keeps you attached to things. It keeps you in a solid box of attachments, and it is called *Mohniya Karma*. The fourth is *Antraya Karma*. This karma can keep good things from being in your grasp and keep blessings from your life. It is one of the major blockages to experiencing good things and prosperity. The last four are not as strong as the former. They are *Nam Karma*, which makes your name popular in either a good or bad way, and it gives you the body and personality type you have. Next is *Gotra Karma*. This karma determines whether a family or dynasty will be well-known and elite or impoverished and bad. *Vedniya Karma* can affect you in two ways: it can bring happiness or unhappiness. The last one is *Aayushya Karma*. This one decides how long you will live in this life.

In review, you now know the five primary sources of collecting karma: body, mind, speech, intention, and mental activities. Through awareness, you can stop collecting karma. Once you do, you can work on the karma already surrounding your soul by doing sadhana, tapas, or *japa* (mantra repetition). In other words, by doing spiritual practices such as fasting. When you stop collecting karma and burn away the old, you will be free one day. Your soul will be awakened. This is the reason you want to fast and work on yourself. You want your soul to be free. Once the soul is free from the grip of karma, it will be awakened. And then eventually, liberated.

How do you explain the reduction of karma scientifically?

Scientifically there is no proven way to explain karma. Scientifically, it can only be explained when we see the result of something, such as seeing bad karma giving a bad result. However, how can you scientifically prove this results from this life or a previous life? There is no way. In the same way, you cannot prove scientifically if you have burned one, two, or ten layers of karma. Science cannot explain everything, but inner realization can.

But the person fasting with the sole intention to wake up and burn karma will know and feel they are becoming lighter and lighter. They will experience going higher and higher. There will be symptoms to prove this, but science is different. Scientists only prove what they decide or hypothesize. Suppose they want to prove that milk is white. The milk is already white, but now they want to prove why the milk is white. They find the logic as to why milk is white. It is already white, so what is scientific about it? An apple is sweet, but now they have to prove the apple is sweet. But that is not scientific. Sometimes I think science is just an absurdity. Why? Because science proves what already exists. They don't prove what they cannot see. They try to ascertain what exists, and people get so mesmerized by it.

The best way to know if karma is reducing within is by fasting and knowing it for yourself. As soon as you begin fasting, you will feel lighter. The heaviness lessens, and you feel different. Later, I will share with you other ways to know how much karma you burn when you fast, but before that, I'll explain a few more things.

How does karma burn when fasting?

Karma burns when your heart and intention is into the fast and not into the food, water, or anything else. When you fast wholeheartedly, the soul awakens. And when the soul wakes up even a little bit, it burns karma. This is the only way to get an idea of how it works. Soul wakes up a little, and karma burns. It burns the endless layers of mountain-high karma. Scientists do not understand karma. Fasting means fire, and that fire burns all the particles surrounding the soul.

How quickly does karma burn in fasting vs. other spiritual practices?

What is interesting about fasting is that if you fast ignorantly, it doesn't burn karma. In Hindu culture, many swamis encourage people to fast. However, they do not know how to break a fast properly. They break the fast by eating algae, and people get fascinated by it. This is considered ignorant fasting because they have no idea that algae contain the most bacteria and living organisms. For your knowledge, if you put your finger in the water under the algae, there are infinite living beings. And if someone is eating infinite living beings, then how are they burning karma? This is called *agyan tapa*, unknowledgeable, or ignorant fasting.

Sagyan tapa is when you have proper knowledge on how to fast properly. When you have this knowledge, fasting will bring a lot of clarity and spiritual upliftment. Why? Because fasting with knowledge is when karma actually burns. You intend to burn karma because you have this understanding that fasting burns karma. Those who fast ignorantly wish to see God, but they can't see God because karma is surrounding them and they have no idea that they should seek how to break it.

I advise people to do tapasya, fasting, with knowledge. Your intention has to be pure. When you fast, you are not fasting for any other purpose other than to burn your karma. In India, girls have a tradition to fast on Fridays so they can get a good husband or get engaged. It is common there. They fast, but they want something in exchange.

They fast for nine consecutive Fridays, thinking they will get a good husband. Other people fast to increase their business also. Know this: you cannot buy a person or prosperity by fasting. Instead of thinking to make themselves pure, they believe they can get something in return. These are not good reasons to fast. Fasting has to be done with a pure intention to burn all the karma, and destroy all the darkness. Fasting with no expectation is the best path.

In spirituality, there are two essential things. One is called *kriya*, and another one is called *gyan*. Kriya is practice and gyan is knowledge. If you have mere knowledge and don't practice it, it will not take you anywhere. Imagine a scholar who collects a lot of knowledge by reading many books but does not apply that information into practice. In the same way, if someone does a lot of practice or rituals without knowledge or understanding it will not take them anywhere either.

I like to give an analogy to better understand this. Suppose a person is handicapped and can't walk and another person who is blind and they find themselves in the middle of a forest fire. One can't walk and the other one can't see, but they both can hear. Alone they cannot escape. But if they work together, they both can get out. The blind man can walk, so he puts the handicapped man on his shoulders and the handicapped man directs the blind man to find the way out. Together they are safe and can escape. Without each other, they would not have gotten far. The same way, mere knowledge is like being handicapped, it will not take you far, and mere practice or rituals is like being blind, it will also not take you far. I do not recommend either alone. I suggest one follows both in sync with each other. *"Gyan kriya bhyam moksha,"* combined knowledge with practice, is a path to *moksha marga* - the path towards liberation. Liberation happens when you remove all the karma, layers, and knots surrounding your soul. You achieve enlightenment when this occurs.

Before you do any spiritual practice, like fasting, gain knowledge before you start practicing. You need both knowledge and practice. But I suggest, first, have knowledge or vision. If you don't have it, don't practice yet. After reading this book I hope you will gain the knowledge needed to understand fasting. Once you understand, you can begin fasting, and you will then reap all the spiritual benefits.

How does fasting compare to other spiritual practices?

Practices like meditation, *dhyana*, are also considered a tapa, a fire. However, the type of meditation that most people are familiar with merely calms their minds down. It works more at the mental level, and it helps to relax their muscles. This allows people to become healthier and more stress-free, but it doesn't help them burn karma. But if somebody can enter a deep meditative state, they can burn mountain-high karma, and if they are fasting at the same time, it will burn very rapidly.

It will depend on how you handle the practices. If you are fasting and reading scriptures that give you spiritual guidance, and suddenly whatever you read hits you deeply, you can burn a lot of karma. Silence is another tapa. It is called *mauna vrata*. Silence alone doesn't burn karma. Silence with knowledge burns karma. There is a lot of discipline involved, and where there is discipline, karma burns. This is why it is important to engage in other spiritual practices while you fast because even little things count and can make a big difference.

When you experience upavaasa, which means you are whole-heartedly into your fast, and you incorporate other spiritual practices, the fire to burn karma becomes much stronger. This is why I recommend engaging in practices such as meditation, yoga, pranayama, Purnam Yoga, mantra chanting, and silence while you are fasting. They will help you even more.

Is fasting the ultimate spiritual practice for liberation?

Fasting is not the ultimate practice. Many great practices lead to liberation. However, I consider it the best one to do if your body allows you. I never recommend anyone fasting forcefully. If the person's body doesn't cooperate, they must break the fast immediately. Do it voluntarily and according to your health. That's the way fasting can help you burn a tremendous amount of karma. But remember, it has to be done with knowledge and wholeheartedly while doing other spiritual practices like meditation, prayer, or chanting mantras. You are supposed to do this, and the fast will be more effective because combined, they work like a fire. It is like adding ghee to the fire, the fire becomes shinier and more powerful, and it burns all the karma, ignorance, illusion, and negativities.

When should we start fasting in relation to karma?

People need a wake-up call. And wake-up calls can happen suddenly because of karma. For thousands of years, it has been that way. Kings from the past would see one grey hair on their head, and they considered it a wake-up call. They would think, "I am going to go down soon. I will die soon, so it is better that I start working on myself more." Then they would renounce their kingdom, leave to the forest, and do a lot of tapasya and meditation to gain clarity. After some time, they would return to share the inner knowing they attained and teach others.

Wake-up calls are many. Unexpectedly someone's body weakens. It used to be strong. So now they may say, "I need to do something with my life. Otherwise, I'm going to die soon." For someone else, sickness or infection attacks their body. Their body begins to ooze. In someone else's case, a beloved one dies, like their own child, and they cannot bear the pain. They ask, "What is this life about? My child died, so that means I will die too." These are all wake-up calls, but people don't understand them.

So, you cannot do fasting until you realize these are all wake-up calls. For example, those girls who fast on Friday because they are so desperate to find a husband see this as their wake-up call. Maybe they started too late to look for one, but this now becomes their wake-up call so they fast. Had they started when they were younger, they might have found the best man. But the problem is that the wake-up call came a little too late for them, and now they are desperate. They are fasting, but their purpose is different. They are not burning karma. A wake-up call has the potential to burn karma, and it can happen to anyone, anywhere, and at any time.

Accidents can happen too. Suppose you lose your leg and you can't walk. You may say, "I'm going to do something about it, I am not going to give up, and I will walk again." You have crutches and begin to move, but later, you find how to get a prosthesis and walk. You do everything you can to rehabilitate and regain full movement. That's a wake-up call, but people usually miss it. Nature always gives you wake-up calls, and that is the time to fast. These experiences should make you realize that life is short. You can lose your body any time, so it is best to work and improve yourself. When this is realized, real fasting begins.

If you are already on the spiritual path, you also get wake-up calls. If your body is feeling heavy and uncomfortable, then it is telling you to fast. It may be because you are eating too much or not eating healthy. You may tell yourself, "Hey, I'm feeling a little chubby, so I better fast." Or you may have too many toxins built up in your system and feel uncomfortable. Spiritual practitioners fast because they realize that their body is the only machine or instrument that can help them achieve enlightenment. When they feel relaxed, happy, and healthy and fast, they can burn a lot of karma. If you are one of them, you don't need to wait to have a wake-up call moment. Take advantage of every day to improve yourself.

What are other factors to determine the best time to burn the most karma?

There are always signals. Signals are when a person feels down or sad. If you feel down or low, then it is time to fast. These feelings suggest that maybe a lot of karma is coming on the way. Those are the symptoms, so fast right away. Fasting helps reduce or burn the bad result those karmas may produce. It can help you be in good shape and not worry about being negative, sad, or unhappy. Even monks fast when they feel lethargic or allergic to the path. Thus, these are signs that indicate you should fast too. And the fast will balance you. Why? Because it is burning your karma.

How can we totally be into the fast and maximize our time while fasting?

As I mentioned initially, fasting is upavaasa. Upavaasa is disconnecting yourself from the instrument that takes you into the world of suffering. What instrument do you have? Christians believe that God gave you this body. The body is your instrument.

It is essential to understand that the soul is weak, and it cannot feel much. A soul that just came out of being algae, for example, will feel nothing. It was asleep for too long. Maybe centuries. Maybe since infinity. That soul that just came out of being bacteria will feel nothing unless it gets a body. It has to be a sensitive body. And a sensitive body is mostly the human body. This is why the human body is very difficult to get. The human body is the soul's only chance to realize the truth and fully awaken. When the soul gets a human body, it means a little karma was removed. Only a little bit, because you may recall I mentioned there are millions or even trillions of karmic layers. And not even one layer of karma out of the trillions was removed when you get a human body. Maybe this is not an exact measure, but I am trying to help you understand that the human body is very difficult to obtain. And once you understand this, it is necessary to disconnect yourself from it. It means your soul has begun to wake up. You understand that you don't want to feed your instrument anymore and that you want to feed your soul more. The soul awakens more and more when you are into the fast.

So how can you get more into fasting? First, through understanding. Understand that you need to remove all the karma surrounding your soul. Whatever it is that is blocking you, you wish to eradicate it. Whatever is keeping you in the dark, you wish to eliminate it. When soul awakens, that person doesn't care to feed the body because their soul is happy. Soul is becoming happier and happier by waking up more and more. Even if you do not feed your senses for one month, the time passes quickly and smoothly. Second, you need to be intensely involved in the fast. When you are too much into tapasya, you will not even remember to eat or be into mundane things. You are totally into your inner self -your soul. When you achieve this, you are doing upavaasa. You reside around the soul more. You are totally into soul.

There is one real example I can give you. A lady in India became very popular. She became a widow in her early twenties. She had no children and was illiterate. After her husband died, she did not want to eat. At first, people understood she didn't eat because of her grieving. For two or three days, nobody minded. But after one week, she still did not want to eat. People were trying to make her eat, but she still didn't eat. People asked her why she didn't eat, and she responded, "What's the point of eating? I loved him so much, and he's not here anymore. What will I eat for?" Incidentally, she got too much into her soul. For years she did not eat. This can happen. It is real but rare. How was she alive? Maybe drinking water or something else, but she survived for years.

This can happen incidentally or by understanding. When it is by an incident, like the widow, you don't burn much karma because the intention is not to burn karma. They don't eat, but their purpose is not to burn karma. People will be mesmerized about their survival without food, but they will not burn karma. This widow eventually came to Delhi to meet me, and I taught her meditation. She had no idea what had happened to her. It is incredible that incidents happen, but they will not necessarily burn the karma unless the person tries to understand it.

When you stop paying attention to worldly things and focus on spirituality, your soul begins to wake up, and it wants to wake up more. This is what it means to get intensively involved. The intention is to burn the karma that has kept you in the dark for so long. Remember this always. You need understanding, intention, and actions to shift towards spiritual doings to free and liberate your soul.

Can confession and fasting remove sins?

People can benefit a lot when they confess what they consider their sins. You can't disclose your secrets to just anyone. It would be best if you found someone you can fully trust and, more than anything, someone who can give you guidance and a penance that can help you dissolve the sin. In the Samanic tradition, we do confession, and fasting becomes the penance. Depending on the confession, you receive a specific penance. Confession by itself can bring much karma to the surface, and fasting becomes a "punishment" to help dissolve it. This penance can be effective only if the person does the fasting wholeheartedly. If they do, it has the possibility to clear and dissolve the karma. That's how it works. It is a system of confession and punishment. However, don't think this system will burn all your karma. Some karmas must give you a result, but it will help you reduce the effect of the karmas when you use this system. If the karmas are small, they can fully dissolve.

Can you burn the karma of a specific sin or bad deed?

You do not necessarily burn a specific karma from your past because you cannot control what specific karmas come up when you fast. In general, they come as a whole. I will explain to you how this actually works. Suppose you collected a really bad karma in your previous life that was supposed to give you a result five lives from now. However, in your present life, your soul suddenly wakes up, and you begin fasting, meditating, sitting in one posture for hours, standing on one leg in a meditative state, or doing other spiritual practices. When you do this, you invite all the past bad karma to come forward and give you a result now. How? Standing on one leg for a long time will create a lot of pain. Right? Your entire leg will swell because one leg is up, and the other one is trying to balance you. I used to stand for eight hours on one leg, and my leg would be swollen and in terrible pain. When you voluntarily submit yourself to these practices, you solicit all the bad karmas, and they come up. Instead of waiting five lives to experience the result of something, by your effort, you accelerate the process to face these karmas. You burn them, and you get rid of them, so they no longer linger.

When you do spiritual practices, you go through voluntary suffering. For example, you are meditating, and you say, "No matter what, I will not move for one hour." And you sit there without moving, not even if a mosquito or a scorpion bites you. All the suffering you endure from it could result from the karma you are inviting and that perhaps, without doing spiritual practices, you would not experience until five lives from now. Why is this good? Because you reduce these karmas' longevity, reducing the number of lives you have to live to free your soul. By inviting karma now, you are shortening your cycle of birth and death so you can liberate yourself much sooner. You do not necessarily invite a specific karma. You invite them all as a whole. They come together as you invite the karma to surface. Be ready for it. That's why fasting requires a lot of courage and strength, not just physically and mentally, but to face the karma that comes up.

Now, there are some karmas that you cannot eliminate completely. They are called *Nikachit Karmas*. You cannot burn them fully, but you can reduce their result by fasting intensively. Similar to what Tirthankara Mahavira had to do. He did intensive fasting and other spiritual sadhana in the forest for twelve and a half years, where he endured so much pain and torture. While he would meditate, someone would put nails in his ears, torture, and curse him. Another person would shout and throw stones at him. And if not humans, animals would come and disturb him too. This went on for many years, but he was always equanimous. He was balanced and never moved while meditating, no matter what infliction of pain he was experiencing. He had to go through this to burn his Nikachit Karmas.

Naturally, when you fast and do spiritual practices, you invite the lighter karmas first. But to access the deeper karmas, you must do deep spiritual practices. You must do intensive sadhana. Intensive sadhana is not a one-day fast. It may be three or five days. You are maybe meditating, not for one hour, but ten hours. Maybe being silent not for one day, but maybe ten. This is how to invite the most severe and deeply buried karma. You have to go very deep and be intensively invested in the sadhana.

You cannot control what karmas surface but bad karma will come up if you are suffering. The more intensive sadhana you experience, the more karma you will burn. Any time is the right time to get started. Everyone is strong enough to take it. If someone can meditate for ten hours, it means someone else can do it too. But people don't want to do it. It means they are weak. I know because suppose a person gets sick and has a wound on the side of their body, and the doctor tells them they cannot change their side. They tell them they have to lay down on the same side for 24 hours, maybe for three days. And for three days, they will not move. So, where did this ability come from? It was always there, but they didn't know it was there, or they just didn't want to do it. But because now they are sick, they have no choice, and they have to do it. This happens with many people.

As another example, the doctor may say you cannot go outside because you just had eye surgery. They order you to stay home with your eyes closed for a few days. You want to see, but you cannot see. But you do it because you have to. You have no choice but to follow the doctor's order. But voluntarily, we do not want to do it. We never say, "For ten hours, I do not want to see anything." But when you don't have a choice, you do it. It means the ability is there, but we don't want to use our power. We have it. Everyone does. And when you use it, it is called intensive sadhana. When you do it, you will sit in meditative state cross-legged for one hour without interruptions.

There are many other ways to burn karma because there are many kinds of spiritual practices. There is not only one kind or one way, but fasting is one of them. And fasting burns karma fast. That is why we call it a "fast."

How much karma can we burn through fasting?

It all depends on how your body reacts to the fast. But upavaasa can burn mountain-high karma in one day. When a person experiences a lot of pain or discomfort, it can burn hundreds of layers. Hundreds, I am talking in one day. This pain can be physical, emotional, or mental. The person may never know exactly how much karma they are burning, but the master will know exactly how much the person is burning. Many knots do not break right away, and the layers are just begging to become loose. Only until you burn a lot will you notice it. Again, the more you are into it, the more that can burn. It depends on the individual.

If we combine other spiritual practices, how much more karma can we burn?

If you are fasting and not doing much, why not meditate, repeat mantras, or do other spiritual practices? If you lie down all day, meditation will never happen. It is best to stay active. If the weather is nice, you can walk around. If there is a road, you can walk a few miles. This will help you get good blood circulation. Afterward, you will get tired, and you can rest. After resting, you can meditate. This process will help you go deeper into meditation. When a person goes deep into a meditative state, they burn a lot of karma.

Spiritual practices, with fasting, can triple the karma burned. If you have little energy, you can also do simple *pranayamas*, like *Anulom Vilom* or *Nadi Shodan*. If you are doing an extended fast, do them slowly. I do not recommend intense breathing because it can disturb your body while fasting. Typically, I tell people to do 700 repetitions of *Kapalbhati* breathing, but I suggest doing a maximum of 300 repetitions while fasting. You can even break the 300 into segments of 100. I also recommend our Purnam Yoga system as it purifies your body even more. Purnam Yoga takes out all the remaining toxins of your body while you are fasting.

Remember that clearing and cleansing your body helps to gain the ability to fast for longer periods. That is how your body, your vehicle, becomes purer. And a pure body helps to go into extended fasting.

What is the formula to know how much karma is burning while fasting?

As I mentioned at the beginning of the book, fasting is not starvation nor something you force. It is upavaasa, which means you stay close to your soul and close to your path. And because you are so much into your soul, you forget to eat or do other things. It means you are wholeheartedly immersed in the fast.

People always wonder how much karma can possibly burn. It is an itch of the mind. They want to make sure that what they are enduring is worthwhile. I will help you understand this by giving you a guideline of different durations of fasts and how much karma you can burn when done wholeheartedly.

The best way I can explain this is to compare it to the karma burned in hellish planets. In hellish planets, people suffer too much. They end up on those planets because of the excessively bad karma they collected. In those hellish planets, people suffer immensely and continuously, moment to moment. Every day they endure torture, and every day they resist it. When they fight it, they cannot burn their karma. Therefore, it only burns as time passes, but time passes very slowly on these planets. Why? Because there isn't a voluntary process there. Someone is torturing them, and they refuse to accept it. In this refusal, not only are they not burning karma, but they also collect even more because all they do is curse, and feel spite and hate towards the person torturing them. The torturer doesn't want to do it, but it is their duty and role on that planet. They both have to go through it.

With this scenario in mind, consider the following formula to get an idea of how much karma you burn in this human life relative to those living hellish lives.

Fast	Description	Karma Burned
Naokarsi	Waiting 48 minutes after sunrise to eat and drink.	The karma burned in 100 years of human life on a hellish planet.
Porsi	Waiting 3 hours after sunrise to eat and drink.	The karma burned in 1000 years of human life on a hellish planet.

Ekasana	Eating one meal once a day in one sitting without moving up or down. You can drink water only before or after.	The karma burned in 1,000,000 years of human life on a hellish planet.
Ayambil	Eating once a day, but only one kind of grain. Like wheat bread broken down into pieces and put in hot water, once dissolved you eat it. No salt or flavoring, nothing in it or added, and you eat it wholeheartedly without resistance. You can drink water during, before, or after.	The karma burned in 1,000,000 x 1000 years of human life on a hellish planet.
Upavaasa	Water fasting. No food intake. Only water for 24 hours.	The karma burned in 1,000,000 x 5000 years of human life on a hellish planet.

Chauvihar Upavaasa	Dry fasting. No food or water intake for 24 hours.	The karma burned in 1,000,000 x 10,000 years of human life on a hellish planet.
Bela	48 hours of dry fasting. No food or water intake.	The karma burned in 1,000,000 x 100,000 years of human life on a hellish planet.
Tela	72 hours of dry fasting. No food or water intake.	The karma burned in 1,000,000 x 1,000,000 years of human life on a hellish planet.
Chola	Any additional 24 hours of dry fasting.	The karma burned in 1,000,000 x 1,000,000 x 10 years of human life on a hellish planet.

There is no other way to compare it because, in these hellish planets, people hardly break karma unless the person becomes really good. They have to tolerate the suffering wholeheartedly without bringing themselves between. Compared to those people, we don't have that much karma because we are not suffering much. The life we have now is considered no suffering at all. To know how much karma we have, we can only see it by knowing how much we can burn in such a short period of 48 minutes. Knowing this helps people to break their karma.

That's why it is best not to collect those types of intense bad karmas that drag you to those hellish planets. It takes forever to burn it, and you experience tremendous suffering. We can break mountain-high karma in our current life on this planet, but we also have mountain-high amounts of karma, like Tirthankara Mahavira. Some say that his karma was the size of the entire Great Himalaya Range with the highest peaks on earth. Enormous mountains everywhere. He had to burn that much. This is why he had to fast for five months and 27 days continuously. During his lifetime, he hardly ate because he had to burn that much karma.

But for you, look at how easily you can burn your karma. In one period of 24 hours of drinking water only, you can free your soul of the karma burned in 5,000,000,000 years of human life on a hellish planet. Eat one meal only once in a day, and you burn the karma of 1,000,000,000 years of human life on a hellish planet. It is your choice how much you want to burn. But can you imagine how much you can achieve if you dedicate your life to purifying yourself?

PART III:

BENEFITS OF FASTING

CHAPTER 8

SPIRITUAL BENEFITS

Many marvelous benefits happen from fasting. Some people believe that you can fast to benefit or help someone else. But fasting only directly benefits you. Indirectly, others can benefit too because of the positive changes you experience and how you heal and transform. Fasting will make you feel better, clearer, and lighter. When you have a healthy body, you have a healthy soul. People don't believe that childhood ever comes back. But in prolonged fasting, childhood returns – you become childlike and pure. Fasting has many spiritual benefits that uplift and awaken your soul, directly improving your well-being and physical, mental, and emotional health. This section of the book will give you a list of spiritual benefits you will achieve by fasting.

The mind and consciousness clear

The mind clears as soon as you stop feeding it. What is the mind's food? Anything that enchants your senses, such as entertainment. Music or lyrics delight your senses. But spiritual music doesn't enchant your senses. It delights your soul. So, it depends on what kind of music you listen to. Sometimes your thoughts can feed your mind. For example, your mind may like a dessert, like Ras Malai, a sweet milk type of dessert, and you think about it. Even though the dessert is not there, you suddenly drool. The mouth waters because the mind remembers it. But when you engage intensively in fasting and other spiritual practices, you don't think of food or even water.

Another way to stop feeding the mind is to repeat mantras. Let's say in one day you are determined to repeat a mantra 10,000 times intensely. You sit or lie down with a pure intention to repeat the mantra this many times. You get so into it so much you forget luxuries and even eating. The more you repeat the mantra, the more the mind gets bored, so it weakens thus giving you less trouble. When the mind loses charge, it becomes an instrument. At that point, the mind becomes your friend and a blessing.

To further understand the mind and consciousness, know that there are two kinds of mind: *dravya manas* and *bhava manas*. Dravya manas is visible or physical. When the mind plays games, it is noticeable. It means the mind is visible. Visible is like having its own patterns, *paryayas*, or its own particles. You can catch it. Dravya manas is like your speech. Your speech has paryaya. It has particles that create a shape or body. That is why you can catch it into a voice recorder. But if it had no structure or particles, you would not be able to capture it. Invisible things you can never catch. But in this case, it is physical and visible. It is not physical like our body, but it is physical enough that an instrument can catch it. And nowadays there are many technologies we can use.

Bhava manas is more subtle than dravya manas, and you cannot see it – it is like a shadow of the soul. It lives close to the soul, and we call it consciousness. Sometimes we use the word soul to refer to it because it is very close to soul. But it is not the soul. However, I consider it the real mind. When bhava manas is involved, there is a pure intention, and if there isn't a pure intention, it is not involved. Why? Because just as soul, when it is too sleepy, bhava manas is asleep too. It is a problem, and it reflects. But if our soul gets a little stronger and wakes up more, automatically bhava manas gets stronger too.

When you fast, that consciousness clears. When it clears, your mind cooperates with you, and whatever you do, it accepts. When you can enter deep into your consciousness, you realize it and experience it. Realization happens only when you enter deeply. How can you enter? Not through the dravya manas – the one that plays games. If the senses are clear, you can then enter into your own consciousness, and your consciousness will take you to the soul. Consciousness is still considered the second mind, but it also gives you access to your soul. But you have to enter into it truly. And it is difficult. Why? Because thieves and intruders are surrounding you. These are the mind and senses, and they are stealing all benefits from you. They have to go, they have to run out, or they have to cooperate with you. Once they cooperate with you, you enter into your consciousness, and then consciousness takes you into the soul. We use the word consciousness and soul as the same, but they are separate.

Dravya manas is always strong. It attracts what it likes only, and it craves things like sweets, fights, hyperactivity, excitement, luxury, pleasures, and desires. But the bhava manas is really pure. To help you understand this, visualize a crystal with a flower in front of it and see the flower's reflection on it. If the flower is red, the crystal turns red. The crystal was clear, but it turned red because of the flower's reflection. Similarly, consider the red flower dravya manas and the reflection of it bhava manas. Bhava manas has no obvious particles or structure like our heart, kidneys, eyes, nose, mouth, and ears do. Even though it has subtle *paryayas*, or particles, they are invisible, like the flower reflected on the crystal. It is just a reflection. It seems to be on the crystal, but it is not. It is an illusion. And that illusion has to go. Your mind is an illusion.

The crystal is like the soul. It is already pure by itself, but it has some color being reflected on it. The color has to be removed because the crystal is already beautiful, and it doesn't need the color. How can you remove the color? By removing the flower in front of it. It means the structure has to go. It means that dravya manas has to be removed. This is how you eliminate it. Once you remove the red flower, automatically, you remove the reflection, the color. And once you do, it releases the soul.

Otherwise, the soul will always be in the grip of both manas. And it is difficult to remove them because people always live in their minds. The highest state of consciousness or soul is a mindless state. It isn't easy to achieve this state. You have to destroy many things; ideologies and beliefs have to be removed. Ideology is part of that reflection. It doesn't exist, yet people get trapped in it. That's why ideology has to be broken. And often, this ideology prevents people from fasting. They create too many ideas about how to fast. They think, "I have to break the fast this way," "I have to have an enema every day while I fast," or "I have to have this kind of food after I fast." They get too involved and sometimes extreme with these ideas. Ideas can be good, but not all ideas are always good. For example, if you do an enema every day while fasting, it will hurt your system. But people have no awareness they are following a wrong idea. That is why I never recommend enemas unless you do it maybe once during the fast to clear your stomach if it doesn't happen naturally. But not every day, but people are people and do it, which is why they get in trouble with their health.

Fasting stops feeding the mind and clears your consciousness. You remove the structure and its reflection so you can live, think, and act from your soul. No reflection is needed. You are already beautiful, just remove the unnecessary, and you will achieve it.

The pranas and energy improve

Prana is life force. The senses are alive because the pranas are there; energy is there. After intensive fasting or intensively practicing other spiritual practices, your energy will be very good. Your energy becomes light. Otherwise, energy is slow and heavy. Sometimes you sit with a person, and you feel heavy energy around you. Sometimes you sit with another person, and you experience a lighter feeling. Why? Because their energy affects you. Their energy is heavy or light. When a person's pranic force is very light, it means they have less karma. Their pranic force is light and clear. When you sit next to that person, you feel peace or experience something unique or different because of their pranic force.

When you fast, your aura also gets affected. Fasting allows it to clear. Sometimes, a person's aura is not bright, but it brightens up when they fast and it becomes clearer. The aura reflects your *chakras*, your energy centers. For example, if someone's fourth chakra gets activated from fasting, their aura's green color will be bright. Automatically when this happens, that person becomes more caring, loving, and peaceful. Fasting helps you to clear your aura too. Clearing means that each color that makes up your aura becomes brighter. All your chakra colors brighten up equally. Intensive fasting and intensive sadhana will give such results.

To do spiritual practices and walk on the spiritual path, you need a lot of energy and strong prana. Fasting increases and clears your energy. Naturally, better energy in your body directly improves your overall mental, physical, and emotional health.

The subtle bodies empty

We have four subtle bodies and together they form our karmic body. Our karmic body is invisible to the naked eye. Although you can't see it, you can feel its vibration. When karma burns, you are emptying that body. It is like a computer chip. If the chip is full of information, you cannot record on it. So, what must you do? You have to empty or delete the information. In the same way, your karmic body has infinite information. In spiritual terms, we call this information karma, and when your karma burns, you are deleting it. When it gets deleted, you can now save some good information in your subtle karmic body. But if there is no space, you cannot store good information.

Good information inspires you. When you lack good information or good karma, it cannot inspire you to do good things for yourself. It's a problem. Nothing will inspire you because there is no space where to store it. People are seeking inspiration, but they are doing it the wrong way. They have to first empty this karmic body. You can learn more about the subtle bodies that comprise our karmic body in my book *Chakra Awakening: The Lost Techniques*. One of the subtle bodies is called the *Tejas* body. It is considered a fire body. This subtle body's function is to process all the karma we collect, and if it is not active, it will not allow you to digest anything. The less karma, the more active it becomes. Otherwise, it is too heavy. But why do we need good karma to be inspired? Good karma gives you a good result. And for people to continue to do good things, they have to see a result. Otherwise, they lose motivation, and they don't want to do anything. The intensity of fasting or sadhana can benefit all areas of your life, making your pranic force stronger, your subtle bodies empty and clear, and your aura more vibrant.

The soul becomes stronger

Naturally, soul strength is one of the most important benefits. When you are into your fast, your soul becomes stronger. It is an automatic process that weakens the mind because you are not feeding it and thus it strengthens your soul. Since you don't feed the mind, you don't feed the senses. The king of the senses is the mind. But you are not eating, drinking, giving it sweets, or anything that fuels it. The act of being deeply involved in your fast or your spiritual practices feeds your soul. The food for the soul is fasting and spiritual practices. It is difficult. When you fast, the first few days are challenging. The mind can give you trouble, but it breaks down after a while and cooperates with you.

The senses clear

Initially, your senses will be bothered, but eventually, they will give up too. Once again, when they surrender, your soul gains strength. But because fasting is not only burning karma, it's burning toxins too, the impact is that the senses clear. Toxins live everywhere in our body, and they plague our minds and senses. Within a few days of fasting, say three days, you have the possibility to remove half a layer. This can help unblock the senses, and when they clear, you can understand the right things through them. When they are not clear, you are more in illusion and confusion, and when this happens, you can go astray from your path. Why? Because the senses become heavier, and you lose control over them. They take you where they want to go, not where your soul wants to go. As you fast, your senses clear, and they become your instruments. They no longer drag you around in the darkness or endless desires. You use them to help you on your path and to help you gain the right understanding of this life.

Karma burns

As you now know, karma surrounds your soul and blocks it from being free. Karma encompasses many things we do not think about. Ignorance, darkness, illusion, anger, jealousy, emotions, negativities, and violence are all part of karma. These are blockages that prevent us from experiencing bliss, peace, and soul freedom. When you fast, you burn these blockages. Your goal should be to stop collecting more karma and burn all the existing karma surrounding your soul. When you burn karma, your soul moves towards becoming a liberated soul, but it will cause an endless accumulation of the same karma that keeps you in the dark if you do not close the sources. The best thing to do is stop collecting karma and take care of all the karma that has built up, obstructing our soul's light. Intensive spiritual practices like fasting will help you burn the karma.

The soul wakes up

When you burn karma, your soul begins to wake up. Darkness disappears. And when darkness disappears, the sun rises. If the sun doesn't wake up, then the darkness doesn't disappear. This darkness is the accumulated karma, clouds, and blockages. Toxins are nothing compared to this darkness. In theory, toxins are a tiny thing. One can remove toxins because they are more physical. But the karma around the soul is like a digital system. It is invisible. And invisible darkness is very difficult to remove. This is why we need intensive sadhana. The whole idea of doing sadhana is to awaken and make our soul stronger. Once the sun rises, the darkness disappears. The soul wakes up, and karma disappears.

If one's pure intention is fervent, it should help wake up one's soul and make it stronger. An example of getting stronger can be like the soul becoming more determined. You become determined about doing something for three or thirty days. It makes you stronger, and once stronger, your soul has no choice but to wake up. Karma has no choice but to run away. You achieve this through intensity, and fasting is no exception. If you are not into it, there will be no intensity. But even without intensity, fasting will burn toxins and can scientifically heal you. If infection, cancer, or sickness is developing in your body, fasting might cure it. Fasting is a preventative measure to avoid disease and the collection of karma. It will help not to bring in new karma, and the old karma will burn. Fasting has a double benefit. It's like having two different desserts in both hands. No matter which hand you taste from, it is sweet. Fasting is like that; it burns toxins, and it burns karma. Both are significant benefits. And most important, your soul wakes up more.

Willpower increases

Fasting increases your willpower. And willpower is needed to grow spiritually. When you have willpower, you can do anything you want. With willpower, you never let distractions and temptations take over you. For example, if you wish to sit in meditation for 45 minutes, you will do it through willpower. If you itch to get up, you will not do it. Even if your body aches, you will not stop. This willpower keeps you going and will help you get through anything. You can survive anywhere in any situation in the whole world.

If you don't have food, water, a place to sleep, and a blizzard passes through, you will survive. Or, suppose an accident happens and a plane gets stuck on an island. The travelers run out of water and food, and they can't locate the plane. In their mind, they don't think they can survive without food and water. Their willpower is so weak, and they die within one or two days. If people's willpower is a little stronger, they can survive for four days, but those with strong willpower might survive 10, 12, 21 days, and I am talking about surviving even without water. But a strong will is needed.

That is the miracle of life. People with strong willpower can fight against anything. They fight with their life, and that gives them a chance to survive. Everyone else will die, but not them. That's why I tell everyone to go through extended water fasting at least once in a lifetime - two weeks, three weeks, whatever they can do. Or do a short dry fast. You can do two or three days maximum. Some people do it, and their willpower increases too.

Intuition becomes stronger

People who are well educated or very intellectual are not necessarily intuitive. Intuition cannot be practiced. It is not a technique or a method applied to something. Intuition merely happens and it can happen to anyone. It is not conditional. It is not known and it does not come from the unknown. It happens to everyone sometimes, but people are not aware of it.

Wisdom comes through intuition. Intuition is the shadow of your soul. It is beyond intellect, beyond mind, and beyond the senses. If we can awaken that, many unknown things will be revealed. Mysteries will be gone. Intuition eradicates mystery because it happens naturally.

When a person fasts, they have the possibility to get totally relaxed. It happens when a person fully accepts the fast. Fully means that the muscles, senses, mind, and everything in you accepts and surrenders to the fast. When this happens, you become totally relaxed. The outcome of becoming relaxed is that suddenly intuition pops up. You might see someone, and out of nowhere, you tell them, "Hey, you are supposed to buy a house." The next thing you know, they buy a house. Or, they might tell someone, "You are supposed to win the lottery today." And they buy a lottery ticket, and they win. They don't know why they say these things, but they cannot resist it. Whatever their first feeling is, they say it, and it becomes true. This is how strong intuition can become.

For this level of power to occur, you must do a long fast. One or two days will not help much. Another way to achieve this is to do another spiritual practice intensively. For example, you sit three hours in a cross-legged position without moving. When you accept the posture, you will become relaxed. If you do not accept it, the mind and senses will be on the way. You will feel pain, and you cannot go beyond it, which means there is no intensity, and if there is no intensity, you will not develop this power.

Experience non-violence in its purest form

No one can avoid violence in its totality as long as they continue to live. It is part of existence. However, when you water fast, you are not putting any food in your body. No food. This minimizes the violence in your life. If a person conducting the fast is a meat-eater, they are not killing animals for food during the fast. Though very minimal compared to eating meat, a vegan and vegetarian diet also produces violence because fruits and vegetables are one-sense living beings. We eat them for survival because they are the lowest category of life and are considered in a coma or "vegetative state." In this state, they cannot feel, which is why there is less violence when you eat them compared to animals who feel pain. When you stop consuming fruits and vegetables, you remove even this lightweight violence from your life.

There are different forms of violence we do not know exist. When you fast, you use the bathroom less. Maybe you are urinating but not eliminating waste material. When you don't defecate, you are not producing anything which can create all kinds of bacteria or living beings. And when your actions don't create living organisms, automatically you reduce violence. So naturally, by fasting, you follow non-violence in many ways.

When you dry fast, you are not putting any food or water in your body. It becomes a higher form of non-violence because there are countless living organisms in the water we drink, so by not drinking water, you avoid this form of violence. You cannot dry fast for too long, but you can try maybe one or two days.

Fasting is an incredible way to reduce violence on the planet. The more we collectively fast, the less violence the world experiences. As you and others burn karma, the energy on the planet changes. When the energy becomes more balanced, the planet becomes more peaceful, and less violence is experienced.

Builds discipline

Inspiration, encouragement, and support can only help you so much to achieve your goals. Ultimately, you need discipline to accomplish your personal and spiritual goals. Fasting allows you to build discipline. There are two ways the mind can be quieted. One way is through discipline, striking it down when it strays. The other way is through bypassing it. An example of a bypass would be when a child who comes home from school turns on the TV and does homework simultaneously. The TV stays on in the background while the child concentrates on their homework.

If bypassing the mind does not work, one requires discipline. Either concentration or bypassing the mind is necessary to enter meditation, and the practice of these methods facilitates the process. When you fast, you build the muscle of discipline, and this discipline helps you to dissolve your mind so you can experience your soul.

CHAPTER 9

HEALTH BENEFITS

There are countless physiological and health benefits when you fast. Many people seek to fast to change their overall health and lose weight. But I always tell people that fasting should be done to burn karma, and in that process, you will automatically benefit physically. Fasting is an integral method of healing and prevention. However, those seeking to change their health through fasting need to consider not only fasting but changing their lifestyle and diet. Stress, eating meat, smoking, drinking alcohol, and anger can make you sick. If someone wishes to change their health but does not improve their environment, habits and lifestyle, they will never have lasting health results post-fasting. A vegetarian and plant-based diet can help you change your health drastically, and if you incorporate fasting occasionally, you will experience even more benefits.

When you are unhealthy, you are prone to disease. What is disease? Disease is your karma, actually. What is karma? As previously explained in one word, we call it karma, but it includes ignorance, illusion, clouds, darkness, all sicknesses, diseases, anything, you name it – it is all included in karma. I will not say that disease is only a health issue. It is a karma issue. Karma is a big concept. If somebody gets sick, it is karma, bad karma. Fortunately, sickness, that bad karma, can be removed and avoided, as you have learned, but it depends on the person's efforts. If they are not ready to put in the steps needed, their health will not change. But if they put in the effort, there are many possibilities. With effort and right guidance, many have healed themselves.

People come to Siddhayatan Spiritual Retreat from around the world to experience both a spiritual and physical cleanse. They love our spiritual retreat because it is situated away from the city in a pollution-free location, and it is very peaceful and supportive. While they fast, they take our retreat classes, chant mantras, walk, practice Purnam Yoga, journal, and spend time reflecting. This environment helps them heal their bodies as they detox. One guest from Michigan had a cancer recurrence. She wanted to experience a spiritual place to fast to heal her body and spend some quality self-care time growing spiritually. She came to Siddhayatan for almost 20 days. She fasted for five days, and then she broke the fast. She ate light vegetarian meals for a few days and then continued fasting for another five. Then she broke her fast and ate vegetarian meals again. She was fully immersed in her fast and experienced a lot of pain, but she pushed through it. She had an intense experience, but in the end, it was worth it. After her fast, she reported to us that the cancer was fully gone.

A young man, in his thirties, came to experience a water fast to heal his body. Five years before he visited, he had gone underwater diving and had issues with his oxygen tank. After coming back up from the ocean's depths, he knew the episode had done something to his brain. From that moment on, he lived with an agonizing headache every single day of his life. For him, it was five entire years of torture, so when he came to Siddhayatan, he was determined to water fast for 40 days to heal his body. On day 38, he broke his fast because all the pain was gone. It was a long and challenging fasting experience, but he did it. His determination and willpower paid off.

One lady had rheumatoid arthritis, and after seven days of fasting, the inflammation in her hands was almost nonexistent. These are just a few examples of things we have witnessed at Siddhayatan, but we have seen many other miracles too. Many people express they feel blessed to have fasted at our retreat and received the support they needed to achieve their goals.

Once, a lady in India called me because her 93-year-old mother-in-law was hospitalized with kidney failure. A Jain nun had visited her and inspired her to take a vow not to eat or drink anything. She told her family it was her wish not to take any form of food or water if she entered a coma. Soon after, she entered a coma, and after three days, she was like a fish without water because even in a coma, a person can feel dehydrated. She had kidney failure, and nothing had worked, so they stopped giving her the water according to her vow. Her grandchildren could not tolerate seeing her in this situation. So, this is when she called me. I asked her what the situation was, and she explained it. She then asked me for permission to break the fast and to give her water. I meditated for a few minutes and said to her, "You will think that I am very cruel, but can you wait two more days?" She said, "Two more days? We thought you would permit us! We thought if at least one of you would give permission, we would be okay to break this vow." I suggested to wait two more days and that no matter how tempted the grandchildren were to give her water, to stop them.

I said this was her will, and if she came out of the coma, she could change her vow. One day passed, and they tolerated it, but the grandchildren couldn't take it the following day. They were taking it moment to moment and going through excruciating emotional pain. They wanted to give her even just one drop of water, but the mother didn't let them. That was the fifth night, and it was a hellish night for them. They couldn't fall asleep. But because I had put a cap of two days, they pushed. The following morning, I got a call. She called me to tell me that something extraordinary had happened. Her mother-in-law had come out of the coma. The first thing she asked for was water, and because she was no longer in a coma, they gave it to her. Later the doctors gave the miraculous news that both kidneys functioned. Both kidneys had healed within five days of not eating or drinking water. This happens when you fast intensively, and you do it when you are aware. She took the vow when she was conscious. Miracles can happen, and it happened to her. She survived because the vow restricted her from taking water, and it burned all the infection, impurities, pollution, toxins, everything, so the kidneys began to function. Sometimes what seems like cruelty is compassion – real help.

What happened to this lady in India is an extreme and rare case. I do not suggest anyone doing this because, in the process, a person can die too. There are no guarantees or predictions in life. Although there is a likelihood of healing, I am not in favor of this. People can lose their lives. Modest intense fasting can heal you too. This approach is a lot safer, and it has tremendous benefits. It not only burns karma and removes toxins, but it can also heal infections, inflammation, problems in the liver and pancreas, and it attacks cancerous cells and burns them all. It heals what medicine and antibiotics can't.

When people fast and die, it could be because there was already too much sickness and damage in their bodies. Whatever condition they had was no longer healable. So, a person may die in fasting, but most people do come out healed. Let us say that if out of 10,000 people, 9,990 come out healed, it shows it's a good system. But who has the courage to do it? That is why I say the biggest addiction is food. People think it is alcohol, smoking, or drugs, but it is not.

Whoever can break the addiction of eating can break any other kind of addiction. Fasting is the fastest way to break any addiction. But they have to go through it. Maybe they have to do an extended fast, maybe a water-only fast. After 30 days, perhaps, their body will become like a baby's body. Their skin becomes very smooth and delicate like a baby's. It is a very good result, but it has to be an extended fast.

As you now know, fasting creates a fire. But the fire needed to heal someone doesn't come in one day. They may need two to three days continuously before they notice inflammation disappearing, infection reducing, or experiencing other benefits. Chronic diseases can be cured, but it depends on the progression and whether people have the courage and willingness to fast.

What are other health benefits we should know?

Fasting is one of the oldest healing therapies. If someone water fasts for 21 days in one year, continuously or in segments, with a balanced vegetarian or plant-based diet, likely they will not get cancer. This combination kills all the cancer cells in the body. You fast for 21 days, which is less than two days per month.

In general, water fasting helps heal or prevent chronic diseases, digestive problems, kidney problems, and cholesterol problems. One of the best benefits is that the pituitary and pineal glands heal. Fasting clears heaviness, headaches, and toxins from the head. If someone has an ear or eye infection, and nothing can heal it, water fasting has a stronger chance.

For people who have a lot of pain in their body or experience cramping a lot, fasting can also heal it. During the fast, the pain and cramps will surface, but it will clear after the fast. A person suffering from chronic pain must fast more intensively to rid their body of the pain. It is a process – a healing process you must go through. The thymus gland, which is near the heart and controls circulation, will function better, and it will help supply all the blood in your body as needed. Fasting is a vital healing process, and people need to know about it. If people follow this system, it can create a miracle in their life.

In general, there is enough evidence backed by science that shows how fasting can aid in these ways:

1. Fights inflammation
2. Improves brain function
3. Boosts heart health
4. Improves metabolism
5. Prevents cancer
6. Improves the immune system
7. Revamps the gut microbiome
8. Contributes to longevity
9. Promotes good health
10. Supports weight loss
11. Protects from obesity and associated chronic diseases
12. Regulates blood sugar levels
13. Protects against and improves conditions such as Alzheimer's and Parkinson's disease
14. Improves blood pressure, triglycerides, and cholesterol levels
15. Repairs and regenerates cells

Can fasting prevent or heal someone from the flu, common cold, or COVID-19?

The flu, common cold, and COVID-19 are viruses that attack the body by spreading throughout the respiratory tract. The person's immune response determines the way the body reacts to the respiratory infection. People with weaker immune systems have a harder time fighting against the virus and may also experience some of the more severe symptoms.

If the person gets a fever, they may not want to eat. A fever is a natural body reaction activated by the immune system to kill the virus and prevent it from multiplying and spreading. Fasting during this period helps to tackle the growing virus. When you have a fever, if you eat, foods can also be contaminated by bacteria and other viruses, so it is best to stay away from other invading organisms. If a person has other medical conditions or severe symptoms, they should only fast in short intervals. Once the fever reduces, you feel better, and you can go back to eating normally.

When someone is sick with any of these respiratory infections, I do not suggest using fasting as a treatment for healing. Fasting should be a preventative measure. Fasting strengthens the immune system and having a stronger immune system allows you to fight any viral infection. It is important to mention, that fasting alone is not enough to build a strong immune system. A healthy and balanced vegetarian or vegan diet, good habits, exercise, a positive environment, low levels of stress, and good sleep are contributors to good health and give a boost to the immune system.

Can fasting cure someone from depression, stress, and anxiety?

Fasting alone cannot heal depression, stress, or anxiety. People who suffer from these conditions will benefit from fasting if they incorporate another system like Purnam Yoga or pranayama. Purnam Yoga and pranayama techniques help to reduce and eliminate these things.

How do we become addicted to food?

Society and parents influence our addiction to food. Because of parents' attachment to their children, they want to give children food and everything else that they want. Why? Because it creates happiness for themselves. They satisfy their own self when they do this. They say, "Oh, this is the best! You will like it!" Yes, the baby will like it because the baby doesn't know anything. Then they give them more. And more. Too much in excess. As an example, children go out on Halloween and collect excessive candy, and they eat it—all of it. And it is all sugar. And sugar makes the children's organs very weak. Parents are supposed to be more disciplined and not give to them so much, but parents have become a little too easy-going. And that is how it all begins.

Since babyhood, parents feed their children processed foods. I understand that life can be too fast. Maybe they are too busy or don't have as much time these days. But the food they are giving their children is not GMO-free, not natural, has too many preservatives, or is overly processed. They don't want to devote the time to prepare it at home and go through that process. Instead, they buy canned food. It is best if parents make the food themselves. That kind of food does not create addiction. Canned food or processed foods do not nourish the body because there are too many preservatives in it. In the long term, it will create trouble. If you occasionally give it to them, it will not affect much when you are truly rushing. But if you give that kind of food daily, it will eventually create addiction and bad habits.

It is already the parent's bad habit to not dedicate the time to prepare fresh, natural, and homemade food due to ignorance or laziness. We spoil children, and we think we are doing a good job by giving them this kind of bad food. No, we are harming their body, their instrument, and their ability to have a strong instrument for their spiritual growth. The baby's body is very delicate and cannot handle everything. Later, as infants or teens, they can get sick, and we think it is genetics, but the truth is maybe we fed them too much sugar in their childhood, which has affected their pancreas, and now they have developed diabetes.

It is like a car. The car needs a little oil to run, but it will overflow if you put too much, and it can damage the engine. Similarly, if you put too much sugar into the body, the pancreas will be overloaded and not function properly. We call this diabetes. Diabetes can be healed if somehow, we can clean the pancreas. There is modern medicine, conventional medicine, but it has side effects. It might assist the pancreas, but it will harm the other organs. Unless in extreme cases, it is necessary. I am not pro medication, modern medicine, or conventional medicine, especially allopathic medicine. Why? Because allopathic medicine always has side effects. This is not the best approach for cleansing. Medication doesn't cleanse you because it adds more chemicals to the body. But if you go through the right process – natural, like an herbal system – then the pancreas might pick up again, but you have to make sure not to overload it further.

When a person grows old, they go back towards babyhood again. In old age, people remember everything they ate in childhood, and that's all they crave. Their childhood returns. If they consumed a lot of sugar or bad foods, that is what they are going to desire. If a person in old age doesn't demand too much sugar and eats a more balanced diet, it shows that their parents raised them with better food habits. It reflects that they are not addicted to sugar or those foods.

However, we live in a society addicted to alcohol, drugs, smoking, sugar, unhealthy food, and bad habits. This is all mental. Why? Because of the mind. The mind reminds you of it, and you crave it. The mind is cunning because it has stored all the memories, and when you hold all the memories, even if the substance is not in front of you, and you say "ice cream," your mouth waters, right? There is no ice cream, but the mind reminds you, and you start craving it, so it shows you are addicted to it. Luckily, if there is no ice cream available, you might not eat it, but if people are too addicted to it and have access to it, they will eat a lot of it. And when they overeat it, they are inviting sickness into their body.

What is addiction? Craving. And to break the craving, you must break the habit of eating food. That is why fasting is the best way to break an addiction. But it will depend on how much damage a person has done to their body. This determines how much fasting they have to do. I cannot tell one person they have to do four fasts because they may have to do 40 fasts – it all depends on each individual. If they cannot fast, they will not break that addiction. But if they can do it, fasting will be the fastest and easiest way to break the food addiction truly, and if they break this addiction, they can break any other addiction.

How else can we avoid addiction?

According to this period of time, people think it is okay to eat three full meals a day. But people need to know their bodies. Sometimes the body cannot handle too much food. Some people know this, and they split their food intake into five smaller meals per day. But it depends on your body's demand. Don't eat unless it is to nourish your body. You have to be disciplined. Sometimes food is available right in front of you, and you don't crave it. Sometimes you are not hungry, but the food looks so tasty that you eat it. But if you are not hungry, don't eat. Test yourself. This is the reason they say, "Eat to live, don't live to eat." If food is in front of you and you control yourself, it shows you are not addicted to it. Simple.

What specific foods create addiction?

Any taste can be addictive, but sugar is the main. But spices, spicy food, salt or any other taste that is developed can create an addiction. Anyone can develop an acquired taste. Like alcohol, it is not a good taste, but it becomes people's habit. Why? Because when they drink it, their body reacts. Maybe their muscles get a boost or relax. But gradually, their muscles get weak. Initially, they feel a boost, like a high. But to flush out all those toxins, they have to drink at least ten glasses of water. If people drink one cup of strong coffee, they will need at least three cups of water to flush it out. Alcohol and strong coffee need to be flushed out. Otherwise, they will create many problems in the body. But people are unaware of this. If you have this knowledge, it is better to be wise and not to drink it in the first place.

How does weight loss happen with fasting?

Weight loss while fasting is natural. The body will burn fat once the glucose in the body gets burned. It is a process called ketosis. Some people don't have too much body fat and are concerned with losing too much weight. However, you only lose weight in proportion to your body. Those who have excess or excessive fat, in general, will lose about one pound per day. If a person's constitution is kapha, they will lose more. There are three body constitutions: vata, pitta, and kapha. I will cover these in more detail in part four of the book, but a kapha body type typically loses more fat during fasting. Kapha is one of three substances we carry in the body, and fasting burns this kapha.

This is important. If a person gains weight while fasting, that means they are making a mistake. They are drinking too much water. Over-drinking will swell the muscles, and then there will be weight gain.

Last, if people have lost weight during the fast but gained much weight after they broke the fast, it means they made a big mistake after breaking the fast. This is why I always say breaking the fast is even more difficult than fasting because when a person breaks, the process of breaking creates more hunger. The cells wake up, and they are hungry, and the cravings happen. People make a mistake to fill up their bellies with everything they used to eat before the fast. They eat all the junk food they crave, and this results in rapid weight gain. In addition, their digestive system can collapse, causing permanent and detrimental damage to their health. If you wish to avoid this, you need to eat small portions of light foods and gradually increase them. Try to have this discipline. I cannot emphasize this enough.

PART IV:

THE FAST

CHAPTER 10

THINGS TO KNOW BEFORE THE FAST

There are many things I have mentioned that could potentially hurt your fasting experience. You have to prepare your body for fasting, especially for extended fasting. Fasting must be done without force, appropriately carried out, suitably broken, and eating the proper foods after the fast. Learn to listen to your body. If you follow these guidelines, your fasting experience will be safe. However, there could also be some adverse symptoms experienced as part of the fasting experience. Be aware that these symptoms could stir up things a bit. Remember, if you don't feel comfortable or safe while fasting, it is best to terminate the fast. A one or two-day fast should not affect you much, but you must always be cautious with extended fasting.

Detoxification can be too much to handle

If a person's body is too toxic, fasting can absolutely be too much for them to handle. It will be challenging, and it can hurt their body. If the body has been toxic for too long, that body has become weak and will not handle fasting. If a person has a hard time fasting, I suggest spreading out the fasts into shorter fasts. If you cannot fast, try a different day. When the environment or weather changes, it might help you. For example, in the winter, a person might have difficulty fasting, but it might go smoother in the rainy season. External factors may help or hurt you. It all depends.

Negativity can surface

You need to know you will likely face yourself during a fast. This is part of the healing and cleansing process. The fast may trigger your emotions and past trauma, and you might experience a significant level of anger. If you are in that situation, you will have two choices: breaking the fast or keep going. You have to evaluate if this release of emotions is affecting you or others. If it is hurting you too much, then you can break the fast and try another day. If you can tolerate it, I suggest you keep going. It is not supposed to be easy, but be at ease knowing you are releasing and burning those emotions. Every day that passes, you will feel it less, and you will feel yourself becoming lighter and less affected from those erupting emotions.

Negative thoughts can attack

Suddenly negative thoughts can attack a person while fasting. This is a natural thing that happens because fasting is difficult, and it can challenge you in many ways. When challenged, negative thinking can take over you quickly. You will be hungry. You may be in pain. Naturally, your thinking changes. You have to be strong and re-shift your thoughts and make them more elevated. Remind yourself of your purpose of why you are fasting. How much you wish to burn your karma. And that will push you through. Engaging in activities always helps. I recommend not to lie down too much while fasting. Keep yourself busy doing what you can do. Those little things will help you not be negative, and time will pass quicker.

Swelling of muscles

This happens when you drink too much water. Instead of healing your body, you will disturb your body. Lack of knowledge can make your body sick. If you are reading books on fasting, I suggest that you only read from those who have gone through the actual experience of long-term fasting. Some people write fasting books and they have not even done fasting themselves. It is like reading a book about swimming techniques from someone who doesn't even know how to swim. Everything depends on each person's situation. You cannot follow those book recommendations because the authors are not knowledgeable enough, even if they are doctors or well-intended. Why? Because their calculations may not apply to you, and their advice may hurt your body. I suggest you drink water according to your thirst. Your body will tell you when you need water.

Health risk

Health risks can also occur by drinking too much water. Usually, when a person does an extended fast, they rest a lot during the first few days. That means the entire body gets a tremendous amount of rest. A person who doesn't have much activity, lies down all day, and drinks too much water, begins to put their health at risk. The entire body, including the muscles and nervous system, can get affected, compromising their health. It is best to stay active and drink water appropriately. Go outside for a walk. Sit under the sun when it's not too hot. Practice meditation or yoga. This will keep you busy and active.

Lack of sleep

During extended fasting, your sleeping patterns change. Your body's system is fully shut down. It is not working a whole lot, so it switches to rest mode. Because it is in rest mode, you may not require too many hours of sleep. Mentally, you may think you need to sleep eight hours a day, but the reality might be that you may only need four hours. I suggest that you stay active during the day as much as your body allows you so you can sleep at night. If your body is tired from the day's activities, you will be more likely to want to rest and fall asleep.

When a person has a cold, they usually rest all day, but they cannot sleep at night. That's why, even if you have a cold, it's better to stay up or take a small nap during the day if you can. This way, you can sleep well at night. Also, if you cannot sleep at night, your mind will be too busy. You will experience too much thinking. And this can serve as an opportunity for negativity to attack.

For those who cannot sleep at night, it is best to fall asleep in the early morning. They will wake up once the sun is up, and they will become fresh again. When they feel fresh and rested, they become inspired to fast another day. The morning brings higher thoughts, and the evening more negative thoughts. Try to sleep at night to avoid negative thinking. Make it balanced and observe your body's symptoms.

What are the three body types and how do they affect fasting?

According to the Ayurvedic system, there are three body types or body constitutions known as the *doshas*. The three doshas are pitta, vata, and kapha. Each constitution has different characteristics, and each reacts differently to fasting. Ideally, all three should be balanced, but often one or two are more predominant. Certain dominating combinations could also put you at higher risk when fasting. That is why it is essential to know your body type to know how your body could potentially react to the fast. A pitta body is more acidic, kapha more mucous, and vata gassier in the simplest explanation. This may explain why some people can easily fast, while it might be a seemingly impossible endeavor for others.

I suggest analyzing and checking your body. If it is too acidic or mucous, it will not be good. If all three doshas or elements are normal, then you can do extended fasting. But even if they are not entirely balanced, you can fast for one or two days with no problem or risk. Almost anybody can do one or two days. However, if they are incredibly acidic, mucous, or experiencing gastric trouble, it is not recommended to fast for too long.

There are online tests or Ayurvedic schools that can help you find out what kind of body constitution you have. You can check. They will give you a test, and according to your answers, they will determine what your dominating dosha is. Some people have a combined result. Both will be dominating, but there is always a stronger one. Whichever is the strongest, that's what I consider the person's body type. However, note which dosha comes in second place because certain combinations are not suitable when fasting. For example, if your primary dosha is vata and kapha comes in second, that is the worst combination. Why? Because the fast will work on burning the kapha, but the gastric trouble will stay in your system, and the gas moves to the brain affecting your head. So, it is best to balance them before fasting.

According to the doshas, the following information will give you a general idea of the symptoms you might experience during the fast.

Pitta Dosha

First, those with a dominant pitta dosha have more acidity in the body. If they try to do an extended fast, they will not be able to. They will have the most difficult time fasting. The acidity will create too much trouble for them, and they will experience too much vomiting and headaches. Unless they remove the excess acid before the fast, they cannot fast successfully, especially long term. If they try to fast, their body will reject it. It will not cooperate. Why? Because fasting creates a fire. And acidity is a fire too. Together they generate more acidity, which can burn your muscles, tissues, and everything else.

There is no medicine to rid this acid. Medication might help to calm it down, but it won't eliminate it. One way to reduce it is to eat more alkaline foods and stop eating acidic foods. This will help to balance it more, but it will still be there. If a person insists on fasting, they can prepare their body 15 days before the fast. They will need to avoid all acidic foods and boost their consumption of alkaline foods. It may allow them to extend their fast by ten days. But if someone wishes to clear the acid fully, the only permanent way to do it is through specific *yogic kriyas*. Yogic kriyas are unique and ancient cleansing techniques. We will teach these kriyas at Siddhayatan. This way, those who seek to remove this acid from their body can have a place to go to and learn how to do it safely. Until then, I do not recommend for them to go through an extended fasting experience. Otherwise, they can risk losing their body. If they force fasting, their body and soul could separate. It means they can die. They can fast, but I recommend no more than one to two days at a time until they clear the acid. And if they fast and feel too much acidity coming up, they need to break the fast.

Kapha Dosha

Second, a person with a dominant kapha dosha is lucky because they can burn the excess kapha or mucus in their body through fasting. However, it will also not be easy for them to fast. They will experience a lot of physical pain. If this happens, they can get a massage to relieve some of it. It is also preferred that they don't do extended fasting. Instead, interval fasting will help them eliminate the kapha, and the more they burn it, the longer they can fast without the physical pain. If they fast with a strong will and push through the pain, they have a high chance of getting healed quicker because of the kapha burning. If too much pain surfaces, it is best to break the fast. Otherwise, they also put their life at risk.

Vata Dosha

Last, those with a dominant vata dosha can fast. Vata is air or gas in the body. Though, if people with this dosha try to do an extended fast when they have too many gastric ailments, they will experience a lot of physical pain and trouble. What happens is, the gas stuck in the body stays in the stomach, intestinal area, and the ribs, and because of the fast, the gas will travel to the brain, and it can make a person go crazy.

It is highly recommended that a person with this dosha avoids foods that create too much gas—beans, meat, potatoes, mushrooms, cauliflower, milk, etc. Before the fast, they should prepare in advance and clear their stomach. Otherwise, the gas will create trouble, especially if they have too much of it. The fast will burn it, but if they can clear their body first, they will avoid the pain and discomfort. If not, the pain will make them very negative during the fast. In general, I suggest getting massages to help their muscles release the gas. While fasting, massage can also help them to avoid the distress.

What are the different types of fasts?

Remember that fasting is the voluntary process of refraining partially or entirely from all food, certain foods, or fluid for a specific amount of time. Fasting is very versatile and flexible to meet your desire and body's ability to fast. For maximum benefits, though, I suggest refraining from all foods and focusing on a water-only fast. It can be done for a few hours to thirty days or more. I recommend dry fasting for a concentrated and shorter fast; no food or water for a limited time for a few hours to a recommended maximum of three days.

To give you a variety of options, I will share with you a list of several beneficial variations of fasting and their descriptions. People think intermittent fasting is new, but it's not. These variations have been a part of the Samanic tradition for hundreds of thousands of years. They have been used with the purest and noblest intent to burn karma. Nowadays, millions of Jain practitioners follow them throughout the year.

Feel free to follow them too and modify them according to your body's ability:

Fast	Description
Chauvihar	Dry fasting - giving up food, water, medicine, or churna (digestive aids) for the entire day, starting from the previous day's sunset to the 2nd day's sunrise. This will be around 36 hours. *For vow use: Chauviharam*
Tivihar	Water fasting - giving up only food for the same length of time as Chauvihar. *For vow use: Tiviharam*
Bela	To give up food and water or only food continuously for two days. *For vow use: Bela Upvasam*
Tela	To give up food and water or only food continuously for three days. *For vow use: Tela Upvasam*
Aththai	To give up food continuously for eight days. *For vow use: Aththai Upvasam*
Masakshaman	To give up food continuously for 30 days. *For vow use: Masakshaman Upvasam*

Ekasana	To eat one meal a day at one sitting and drinking water as desired between sunrise and sunset. *For vow use: Ekasanam*
Beasana	To eat two meals a day in two sittings and drinking water anytime between sunrise and sunset. *For vow use: Beasanam*
Sudh Ayambil	To eat once a day, one meal containing plain boiled rice without salt, flavoring, or spices, and have water in one sitting. Nothing else is permitted. Water can be taken any time during the day, starting at 48 minutes post-sunrise and before sunset. *For vow use: Sudh Ayambilam*
Thamb Sudh Ayambil	To eat once a day, one meal containing plain boiled rice without salt and spices, and have water in one sitting only. Nothing else is permitted, and no water after the one and only sitting. *For vow use: Thamb Sudh Ayambilam*

Ayambil	To eat once a day, one meal containing only boiled or cooked grains free of spices, salt, milk, yogurt, ghee, oil, oilseeds, vegetables, fruits, sugar or anything else. It is plain and tasteless cooked grains. *For vow use: Ayambilam*
Navkarsi	Food and water are consumed at least 48 minutes after sunrise. *For vow use: Navkarsim*
Porsi	Taking food and water after 1/4 (25%) of the day passes. Approximately three hours after sunrise. *For vow use: Porsim*
Sadhporsi	Taking food and water after 3/8 (37.5%) of the day passes. Approximately four hours and thirty minutes after sunrise. *For vow use: Sadhporsim*
Purimuddha	Taking food and water after 1/2 (50%) of the day passes. Approximately six hours after sunrise. *For vow use: Purimuddham*

Avaddha	Taking food and water after 3/4 (75%) of the day passes. Approximately eight hours after sunrise. *For vow use: Avaddham*
Varshitap	To eat on alternate days and water fast on the rest, for a whole year. This fast is very difficult as it requires an entire year's commitment to eat on alternate days and eat no food on the rest of the days. *For vow use: Varshitap Upvasam*
Unodar	Eating less than your desire and to simply avoid hunger for your chosen length of time. This is considered a partial fast. *For vow use: Unodar Upvasam*
Vruti Sankshep	Limiting the number of items eaten for your chosen length of time. *For vow use: Vruti Sankshep Upvasam*
Rasa Parityag	Giving up your favorite foods for your chosen length of time. *For vow use: Rasa Parityag Upvasam*

Olee	For 9 days eating simple foods without added flavors such as oils, butters, ghee, salt, sugar, spices, etc. *For vow use: Oleem*
Phal	Giving up all food except for fruits. Water can be used in moderation throughout the day. *For vow use: Phal Upvasam*
Shakahari	Giving up all animal products and their derivatives, including meats, eggs, dairy, and honey. Eating only fruits, vegetables, beans, nuts, and whole grains. *For vow use: Shakahari Upvasam*

How can one determine the number of days to fast for?

People ask this question a lot. They want to know how long they need to fast to heal and cleanse their bodies. There is no precise number for everyone because, as you understand now, many aspects influence fasting. The level of stress, number of toxins, diet before the fast, your current environment, physical and mental health, body type, and food eaten right before the fast are all factors that affect the fast. A person may want to do 30 days, but their body may let them do two weeks only. A person with too much acidity may have to end their 14-day fast after five days. So, you never know. However, if this is your first time fasting, I suggest starting with one to three days.

Some people have never done fasting before, and they jump straight into a 30-day water fast, and they are successful in completing it. Maybe all the conditions were in their favor. I suggest to take it day by day. You can have a general idea of your target, and you can push yourself to achieve it, but when it feels forced, it's best to interrupt the fast and break it.

In general, for a first-time faster, under the right conditions and elements, one could fast for five to seven days. I always tell people that the real fast begins on the fifth day. After day five, the fast begins to purify your body and soul truly. This is how long it takes to hit the deeper layers of karma. Don't be discouraged if you can't last for five to seven days straight. Remember, you don't have to fast consecutively; you can spread out the days. If your body and mind cooperate with you, keep going after seven days, try to reach 14, and keep going if you can. I always recommend everyone to at least once in their lifetime experience a long, extended fast if their body allows.

You now have several options of fasting variations. If you cannot do one month of drinking water only, try to do Ekasana or Beasana for one month. There are many other combinations or options you can try. There really should be no reason for you not to try at least one kind of fast. It is up to you how much you desire to heal your body, clear your mind, improve your health, and burn your karma. Whichever fast you do, do it wholeheartedly and with no expectations.

How many days of fasting will it take to burn toxins?

If a person is full of toxins, they will have a hard time fasting, so they have to go slow. I suggest they try fasting for three to four days, and if all goes smooth, then they can continue. After day five, they will burn many toxins. In the first four days, they burn approximately two layers of toxins compared to 41 days of Purnam Yoga alone. Remember, these are layers of *toxins* and not layers of karma.

If you incorporate Purnam Yoga or pranayama breathing techniques, you can increase the number of layers of toxins you burn depending on how much of it you do during the fast. The results can triple. You would have to do two to three hours of it to triple the benefits. A guest who came to Siddhayatan from London got rid of his cancer. He was fasting, doing two to three hours of Purnam Yoga daily, and following all the teachings I taught him. The doctor had given him only five months to live, and it has been four years since he came, and he is still alive. The cancer was stage IV. Miracles like this can happen when you are intensively involved with both.

What is the maximum time one should fast for?

A person needs to be careful about how much and for how long to fast. Remember that fasting is an open invitation for karma to surface and give you a result. Be modest when choosing the length of time. Don't compare yourself to other's experiences, nor compete either.

One student from California came to see me because he wanted to fast. He wanted to fast for 30 days, but I suggested for him to do only 8 days. He did not listen to my advice and he completed the 30-day fast. Why I didn't support his idea to fast for 30 days had nothing to do with his body's ability to fast. It concerned the karma, which I saw he had, that could potentially surface if he did.

He safely completed and broke the fast. However, a few months after breaking the fast, he was driving during the night around 2:00 am, and he got into a major car accident. It was a hit and run, and his car was totaled. Unexplainably, the police found him out of the car on the road unconscious. He was taken to the hospital immediately with many broken bones, including the backbone.

He was in a coma for a long time and I visited him a few times at the hospital. I suggested that his family play a specific type of music and told them I felt he would come back. He took six to eight months to come out of the coma, but he finally did. The comeback was not pleasant. He returned to his life, but he was now disabled. He couldn't work and his wife had never worked before, so he was in a very difficult situation. With time and effort, he slowly improved his life and physical condition and now he can walk and partially work.

His intention was pure. He was knowledgeable about using fasting to burn karma so he wanted to burn his karma, but he invited all this trouble that followed the fast. It was the consequence of his karma. The karma he experienced was supposed to appear ten lives later, but his fast brought it much sooner. This process is called *udirna* --

the result of karma appearing prematurely. He was fortunate to not fully mess up his life. He could have lost his life had he done more fasting. Nowadays, he still does his sadhana and when he asks about fasting, I only suggest for him to fast one day here and there. Now, he listens.

The karma you invite can appear during the fast or even after the fast. This is one example of why I always say to be careful with fasting. Even though you are burning the karma, the result can become too much to handle. Even if a person's body can handle a long fast, it is unknown what karma will appear. Scientifically speaking, a person's body can water fast for up to 90 days. After that, it can be a significant risk. There are always exceptions. It could be rare that a person can fast further. But in general, with the physical body we have and a strong willpower, we could go for about 90 days. That is, if the body is still digesting the water and not throwing up. Tirthankara Mahavira fasted for almost six months, but his body was exceptional. His body was powerful and different.

In terms of dry-fasting, I suggest a maximum of eight days. Again, this is only if a person's body can tolerate it, but typically I don't recommend more than three days. For all other fasts, go to the maximum time your body and mind can handle. Be modest with the duration of your fast. Take it day by day, be flexible, and never force it.

What kind of water is best to drink while water fasting?

In one glass of water, there are almost one million living beings. When there is considerable water, we call it a body of water. But it is an accumulation of countless living bodies, and together they form the ocean, a lake, a pond, or a river. Among these living beings, you will find good and bad bacteria, viruses, and parasites. Our body needs the good and healthy bacteria for survival. However, if the water is not treated properly, those harmful bacteria, viruses, and parasites can enter our body, creating endless health problems. For example, if you use or drink contaminated water with certain strains of E. coli, you can get food poisoning, pneumonia, urinary tract infections, diarrhea, to mention a few. And they can lead to life-threatening symptoms.

In fasting, this is why I always suggest not to drink water as it is, coming directly from a river, stream, lake, or well. Within 48 minutes of pulling it, many more bacterias will be born. You never know what living organisms are found in the water, and you might not be able to digest them, or they will reproduce in your body, creating problems for you. This is why it is important to boil the water first. Let it cool down, and then you drink it. It will kill all harmful bacteria, and you will be better off. This is the kind of water I only drank during my 32-day water fast. It is safer because there are fewer chances of bad living organisms going into your stomach because the heat kills them. After the water cools down, it takes hours to grow millions of bacteria again, so it is preferred to have a filtration system for further protection. I suggest, personally, to only drink clean, purified, and treated water.

If you are fasting for one to three days, it doesn't affect what kind of water you drink, as long as it is purified and plain. For extended fasting, though, I recommend that it has to be fully treated. I do not suggest bottled water, because you don't know if it is old water or contaminated by the plastic. It is best to have purified and natural water, but don't trust outside sources. Water can come with impurities and harmful bacteria, even in bottled water. You never know. Sometimes companies cheat, so they are not trustworthy. In India, they boil the water and let it cool down. Once it is room temperature, they drink it. This water is less risky. I think it is best to treat your own water; either boil it or use a high-quality filter that can take all the impurities out.

Many people believe that the best water to drink during an extended fast is distilled water. But I will not suggest drinking distilled or reverse osmosis water. Distilled water is when you boil the water into steam and condense it back into liquid in a separate container. Reverse osmosis removes minerals and ions from the water. Both methods strip away all the minerals from the water, and when you drink it, your body will not replenish any of the minerals lost from perspiration. Regular filtered water takes out all pollutants, impurities, and harmful bacteria, but it keeps the minerals. However, if you still wish to drink distilled or reverse osmosis water for a couple of days, you can do it as it will not affect you much.

But carbonated mineral water or sparkling carbonated water is full of minerals. It is also not recommended during a water fast because you get too many nutrients, turning your fast into a partial or limited water fast. It is not considered a real water fast. The body's system will get confused after a while. It will not know if it is shut off or not. This water doesn't allow your system to entirely shut down because it is full of minerals, nutrients, and sometimes, sweeteners and flavoring. You will not get the deep benefit you are seeking – it will not surface the karma, and you will not burn it.

What should one know about the water consumed while fasting?

The water's temperature also plays a role in fasting. During a long fast, I do not recommend cold or icy water. It is not good at all, because your body's system is shut down and cold water is not good for it. Why? Because it can take up to three hours to digest it. This means that your body has to work harder to process it. Also, the body internally is warmer due to the fast, and drinking cold or icy water can shock it thus, why I do not recommend it. It is best to drink warm or room temperature water. If it is cold outside, hot water is acceptable if you sip a little bit at a time.

How much water should be consumed?

These days there are many misconceptions about how much water to drink during water fasting. According to doctors or so-called "fasting experts," you need to drink liters or gallons of water. When fasting for one or two days, it will not make much difference in how much water you consume. But in extended water fasts, over drinking water can lead to intoxication, resulting in debilitating health conditions. When too much water is present, it dilutes the levels of sodium and electrolytes in the blood. When this happens, the cells swell, swelling the brain, muscles, and organs. Overhydration creates similar symptoms to dehydration, so be aware that this can include headaches, nausea, vomiting, and diarrhea. If at any time during the fast you experience these symptoms, check the level of water you are consuming and cut back if needed. If the symptoms persist, break the fast. Other signs you are drinking too much water are not losing weight or gaining weight while fasting.

So how much water should you drink? You need to listen to your body. Thirst is the best indicator of when your body needs water. The level of activity you engage in, the weather conditions, environment, how much you perspire, and your overall health will determine how thirsty you get. When you are in tune with your body, you will know if you are drinking enough or not enough water. Drink adequate amounts, but gauge it to ensure you are not dehydrating or over-hydrating yourself. If you feel like you are forcing yourself to drink water, it already shows you are overdrinking.

Where should people fast?

If you have a strong will, you can fast anywhere. If willpower is weak, it is best to go to a place where you depend on others and where you cannot get food from, like a spiritual retreat or a natural place. You cannot get food at such sites, at least not easily, and you will not be as tempted to eat. If you stay home, you might have a harder time.

There are many temptations; you will have easy access to food, you might have to cook for your family or watch them eat, you might watch television and see all the food commercials, or you might drive by and smell all the scents from the restaurants enticing you to eat. When you go to a retreat, you are far from temptations, which can lead to impulsive eating. Many people are very strong, and they have a strong will, so they can fast no matter where they are at. However, the environment around them will affect their fast.

Why is the environment important for fasting?

The environment affects fasting. If you are full of stress, worries, tension, or are too busy, you cannot relax enough to let your body heal and take a total break. The best environment is a place free of pollution, stress, negativities, and is as natural as possible.

Most cities are polluted, and if you are doing an extended water fast, you are inhaling those pollutants. This is not good because your body becomes purer as you fast, but they can attack you if these pollutants enter your body. That's why I suggest going far away to a natural place like Siddhayatan where there is no pollution. Our retreat is simple and in nature. Fewer cars are driving by, less pollution, no televisions, and few distractions. Television can become a significant influence on your emotions. If you are watching bad news, you will get angry. If you watch violent movies, you absorb that violence. When you purify yourself in a place where you are watching the news or bad things, those bad things will attack you, and your fast will be ruined. Remember what I said before, fasting is upavaasa, and upavaasa is staying close to your soul. Be wise to choose the location and environment for your fast.

An ashram helps you set the deepest intention: to burn all the bad karma blocking you. Bad karma makes you wander in the dark, blocks you, and keeps you depressed, anxious, and in illusion. At an ashram, you can learn ways to heal further and grow spiritually. That is why we developed and teach our Purnam Yoga system at Siddhayatan. You can do it in addition to fasting. Together, it deeply purifies the body and helps bring a person out of depression, anxiety, and panic attacks. There is no one way to do fasting. You can always do more. When you combine these techniques, you might double or triple the benefits.

There is a saying in India that says, "In a cup of milk, you put one spoon of sugar, and the milk tastes better. You put two spoons of sugar, and it tastes even better." When you add sugar, it makes it taste sweeter. If you put half a spoon, it will not be as sweet. In the same way, if you only fast, it will not be as sweet as if you added a spoon of intensive Purnam Yoga, meditation, mantras, or silence.

How does the weather affect fasting?

Weather, to a great extent, can affect fasting - positively or negatively. There are places on the planet where it is mostly somber; countries like Finland, Norway, or Estonia. These places get only a few hours of sunlight. Sometimes they don't get any sunshine at all. It is very depressing. That's one of the reasons why many people that live in those countries are depressed. Even when it is daytime, it is cloudy, and you cannot see the sun. People who live too much in the dark become too depressed. The more people fast in these places, the more help they will receive. They become more stable because the fast allows them to burn their karma, and if they go deeply into their fast, they can burn substantial amounts of karma.

There are places like Texas, where you mostly experience sunny days. Good weather can benefit fasting because the body likes sunshine, and fasting becomes easier to do. They will burn karma because the fast is going well. But easier fasting doesn't always equate to more karma burning. In fact, people will not burn as much karma as those who live and fast in darker places.

If it rains, it will have a greater positive effect when dry fasting. When it rains, all the pores absorb the moisture or humidity from the rain. It is good because you do not get as dehydrated, and the fast can go more calmly and peacefully. It is a good idea to dry fast during rainy days. While in tropical weather, though, if you are water fasting, you cannot drink too much water because there is already too much moisture in the air, which your pores will absorb too. This can create the problems I've mentioned before about drinking too much water while fasting. But if you are in a dry area like Arizona or the desert, you would need to drink a lot more water. You might be tempted to drink cold water in a hot climate, but as a reminder, I recommend drinking room temperature or cooled-down water after boiling it.

Fasting in extreme temperatures will not be as easy, but nowadays, many people have a controlled climate in their home. We can sit inside our home and be comfortable when the temperature outside is 110 degrees. But that is not the real fast. The real fast happens when you are in a more natural climate. You can fast when the weather is more tolerable so you can be in nature more. That burns the real karma. Why? Because you are in nature and not in luxury. I am not saying that if you fast at home, you will not burn karma. It will still create a fire. It will still burn karma, but the results will vary. You will not burn as much as you could have by fasting in a more natural and simpler environment. For example, if you are fasting at a medical clinic with doctors, you will not get the same result as fasting in nature or at a spiritual and simple place.

How does the moon impact a fast?

The moon is responsible for the low and high tides of the ocean. In the Samanic tradition, we teach that you will be affected by the full moon if there is too much water in the body. The body comprises 70 percent water, so you can get affected when you do a water, juice, or fruit fast.

Since fruits and vegetables can have up to 90 percent water, you can become overly emotional and experience drastic mood swings. That water is condensed. It is so concentrated that if you eat many vegetables and fruits, it is like adding an additional 20 gallons of water, even in one meal. Condensed water can be too much, and the full moon will affect you. That's why the Samanic tradition says not to eat fruits or vegetables during a full moon, only eat dry foods, even if you are not fasting.

Dry foods are things like beans and grains. They have only the water you use to cook them with, so they will not affect you as much. Most people do not have this knowledge, and they eat the wrong foods during the wrong time. The Samanic tradition follows this system. The Samanic tradition, since the beginning, has focused on spiritual growth. The physical and mental healing that occurs is a byproduct of it. That's why I suggest fasting for spiritual growth, and no matter what, you will experience physical and mental cleansing.

CHAPTER 11

PREPARING FOR THE FAST

Every fast is different. Several factors affect the outcome of your fast, two being the condition of your body and the foods you eat before the fast. If you prepare your body and clear your stomach, the fast will go a lot smoother. You can do an enema to clear the colon. However, that is a forceful and unnatural method. No matter if you are fasting for health or spiritual reasons, it is best to prepare your body beforehand. Consume more fluids, juices, and soups. Within two days, the stomach will flush unwanted waste material stuck in the intestines, and the fast will go smoother. If smoother, negativities will not surface as much. If people don't prepare adequately, they will experience pain and discomfort, which generates a lot of negativities. It is best to prepare to have a smooth and more consistent experience when fasting.

There is a misconception that the fast will clear the body. But it doesn't work that way. You have to clear the body first so that the fast can fix your body. Empty the stomach, and you will have an undisturbed experience. When waste material stays in your system, it creates the gas that travels to the brain producing headaches, heaviness, and negativity. And the mind lives in the head, so imagine the burden it will create for you.

What is the best way to prepare for fasting?

One of the essential things you can do before you fast is to empty your stomach, especially if you are doing it for a more extended period. Emptying the stomach means ensuring your last meal gets fully processed and digested. You can accomplish this by consuming a more liquid diet or very light foods two days before the fast; this way, your stomach and intestines will not have to work too hard to break it down. Examples of what you could eat are fruits, vegetables, soups, smoothies, juices, and water. They will digest quickly within four to six hours.

Some people have the misconception they need to stuff themselves before fasting. They think they have to eat a lot so they can survive the fast. But they have the wrong idea. Never fill yourself up before a fast. Prepare two days before; this way your long fast will go smoothly. Even if you are fasting for two to three days, I still suggest that you prepare one day before accordingly.

When heavy foods are consumed, they sit longer in the stomach.

When this happens and you are fasting, it can create complications in your body. Things that can occur are:

- Sickness
- Headaches
- Acidity
- Indigestion
- A burning sensation on your chest and throat
- Gas, which can travel to brain, making you dizzy and unstable
- Risk of migraines
- Make your tongue smell
- Bad breath

Foods or ingredients that are heavy, toxic, and difficult to digest are meats, unhealthy starches or carbohydrates, fried foods, alcohol, caffeine, and highly processed and canned foods. Two days before, avoid these foods, including acidic, gassy, and mucus-producing foods based on your dosha.

If you are constipated, do not fast. Wait until you can clear your stomach. It is preferred that you find a natural way to go to the bathroom, but if nothing works, you can take a laxative or use an enema, but do not consume food after. Try not to do an enema in the middle of the fast. Otherwise, you might be taking a risk. If you need to do one, do it before you begin the fast.

When is it ok to skip the preparation process?

I recommend that everyone follows the preparation process. Sometimes, if a person has too much acidity, such as those with a pitta dosha, they have to prepare 15 days before by reducing and eliminating acidic foods.

In cases where the person is totally healthy, doesn't have sickness, has balanced doshas, or doesn't have constipation, they can start the fast without preparation. If you are fasting for just a few days, one to five days, preparation is preferred, but you will not experience much of the symptoms I've described if you don't prepare. For anyone fasting beyond five days, I strongly suggest the preparation method I mentioned. If a person struggles too much during the first few days, it shows their stomach was not empty.

To prepare, follow the next set of recommendations:

- For extended fasting, prepare at least two days before.
- For short fasting, prepare at least one day before.
- Consume more light foods and liquids.
- Make sure your stomach is empty.
- Eat primarily vegetables, fruits, soups, nuts, smoothies, water, juice.
- Avoid heavy, toxic, and acidic items such as meats, alcohol, caffeine, spicy foods, fried foods, unhealthy starches, junk food, processed foods, and heavily seasoned foods.
- Do not eat in excess.

- For acidic bodies, 15 days before an extended fast, eat more alkaline foods and eliminate acidic foods.

What is the importance of taking a fasting vow?

In the Samanic tradition monks, nuns, and laypeople take a vow or oath before they begin a fast. We call this a *pachakhan*, which means "oath" in Sanskrit. The oath is repeated with folded hands and it is taken by the witness of an *Acharya*, a spiritual leader, *Siddha*, liberated souls or God, *Arihanta*, an enlightened master, or *Guru*, spiritual teacher. Anyone can take this vow from anywhere because at least one of these divine beings is always present. Even if you do not have a teacher or if they are not available, Siddha or God is always present.

People are bound by their mind. When you take a vow, you prepare mentally that you will not break your fast no matter what happens. You take the vow according to the type of fast you've chosen. When you take it, you do it in the presence of God or Guru, so you don't want to insult them by breaking it. The vow helps you create discipline for that period making you stronger and more capable of completing your fast. If you don't take the vow, you are free. There is no commitment, so you might get weak and eat. But if you take the vow, you will not eat. You can commit to not eat anything for one day, and for 24 hours, a person can survive easily.

The vow has to be taken daily according to the number of days one wishes to achieve. When you fast, you fast one day at a time, gauging if it is safe to continue. If fasting, you may want to consider taking a vow to strengthen your purpose and commitment to the fast.

How does taking a vow affect the fasting experience?

Taking a vow makes you totally disciplined. Fasting helps you follow the *samyam*, the discipline, and samyam burns your karma. Most people are mentally weak, but if they take a vow they might stick to their intention. When you don't take a vow, you might not complete your fast. Therefore, taking a vow will affect fasting because it will help you achieve your goal.

Will more karma be burned if one takes a vow?

Taking a vow is more of a mental preparation. Whether you take a vow or not, if you complete your fast you will burn the same amount of karma. However, not taking a vow can derail you. I will give you an example. If a layperson is living life like a monk, but they never took the vows of a monk they will not burn as much karma as the monk, even if they live their lives exactly as the monk's. Why? Because the monk took the lifelong vow that no matter what happens or what they go through they will stay on the path of helping themselves and others. That is how a vow works. Therefore, even if a layperson or householder is doing more spiritual practices than a monk, they are still not at the same level because they never took a vow. Why? Because they are not bound yet. They are not disciplined yet. They go out here and there, they see ice cream in the market and they will eat it. Their weaknesses are on the surface. The temptations are there.

When you take the vow, there is no temptation. Those without a vow can go astray any moment. They can get tempted. Thus, when you take a vow there are no temptations. Taking a vow guarantees you will achieve your goal and burn the karma.

What happens if you break the vow by mistake or intentionally?

When you break the fast by mistake and you become aware of it right away, it is not considered breaking the vow. By mistake, it is forgiven. If you take the vow and you get sick, you must request permission from your spiritual teacher or whoever gave you the vow, this way, you do not collect bad karma. However, if you break the vow intentionally then you collect a lot of bad karma. Never break your vow intentionally. If you are wavery about fasting, it is best not to take a vow in the first place. Here, you are better off by not taking the vow, otherwise, instead of burning karma, you collect more. Why do you collect karma? Because you take the vow in the witness of God, Guru, or Acharya and if you break it, then it means you don't respect them.

When a person doesn't respect anything, especially God, they will not care if they break a vow. So, if you are unsure, don't take it. Be free from this worry. Just decide what you wish to achieve and be determined to complete it.

What are the benefits of taking a vow?

Remember that a vow puts you in the samyam, in the discipline. Discipline is a voluntary process that no one is forcing you to do it, and it burns a lot of karma. When someone forces you to do something, you do not burn karma. For example, if a correctional officer forces a prisoner to stand in the sun for four hours as a punishment, that person doesn't burn karma. Instead, they collect more because they resist it and they build anger, hate, and animosity towards the officer. But if a person voluntarily stands in the sun without moving for one hour, they will burn a lot of karma. A vow is voluntary out of your own free will, it is not forced upon you. You take it to have discipline and strength. Exceptions are everywhere, so if there is sickness or the person's health is not good, they can break it with permission.

What vow can be taken from anywhere?

At Siddhayatan, I give my students a special vow when they fast. Taking the vow inspires and motivates them. They also express it brings them closer to the experience of upavaasa, residing closer to their soul, during their fast. You may also take it if you wish to strengthen your commitment to your fast:

ARIHANTA SIDDHA ACHARYA GURU SAKSHI BHAVEN, UGGAYE SURE NAMOKAR SAHIYAM _____ PACCHAKHAMI SAVVA SAMAAHI VATIYAAGAREN, APANAM VOSIRAMI.

The general meaning and interpretation is:

By the witness of Arihanta, Siddha, Acharya, and Guru, to the next

sunrise and reciting the Namokar mantra, I will complete the
_____ fast, with the only exception to break it if my
body feels ill. I take this oath with my soul and stand firmly with it. In
the line, fill up the name of the fast you've chosen to do. Go to pages
176-180 and refer to the "for vow use" line. Then, when it's time to
break your fast, recite the Namokar mantra three times with hands in
prayer position over your heart:

Namokar Mantra
Namo Arihantaanam
Namo Siddhaanam
Namo Ayariyaanam
Namo Uvajjhaayaanam
Namo Loe Savva Saahunam
Eso Pancha Namokaaro
Savva Paavappanaasano
Mangalaanamcha Savvesim
Padhamam Havai Mangalam

Pronunciation
Na-mo Uh-ri-han-taa-nung
Na-mo Sid-dha-nung
Na-mo Eye-ya-ree-ya-nung
Na-mo Uva-jay-ya-nung
Na-mo Lo-e Sa-va Sa-hu-nung
Eso Pan-che Na-mo-ka-ro
Sa-va Pa-vap-pan-na-sa-no
Manga-la-nung-che Sa-ve-sing

Pada-mung Hav-eye Manga-lung

To take the vow online or to hear the vow and Namokar pronounced properly, visit https://thefastingbook.com/vow.

CHAPTER 12

WHILE FASTING

It is better not to have expectations during a fast. What I mean by that is don't expect a specific result or type of experience. Remember, the benefits will be many, but most importantly, you will burn your karma. What is essential, though, is to be educated about some of the things that may occur during a fast. You cannot predict each person's experience because it will be different every single time. Some fasts may go very smoothly, while others might bring many difficulties. But in general, trust this process of burning karma. Follow all the recommendations, and don't force fasting.

I will share with you some everyday things you may experience while water fasting along with some guidance. Read all the symptoms because, for some, the symptoms may come up sooner.

First six days

On the first day, typically, you do not feel the absence of food too much. On the second day, food thoughts will attack you. It becomes mental because you've consciously decided to drop the food. The third day can create pain in the body, uneasy feelings, and headaches. The headache typically stops on day four because when you don't eat and drink only water, the headache has no place in the body. It has to end or at least diminish by then. These feelings reduce or fully clear on day five or six.

These symptoms may be experienced by many. In my case, I had body pain everywhere throughout all my muscles. It was only until the sixth day that my real fast began. My body became light, and the pain cleared – the real fast began. When the person's body settles or becomes light, that indicates when the real fast begins. When this happens, you will feel your energy coming back.

Many people cannot handle five days or have the time to fast for this long. Typically this is the hardest part, but afterward, it tends to go more smoothly. Many people break the fast before they reach this point, in many cases, because they have to return to work. I suggest that you take time off from work. You never know where your real fast may take you. You might be able to complete ten days or maybe even two weeks. For those who can do it, it is good to have this experience.

After the real fast begins

Generally, the fast goes smoothly after day six, but once you get to around day ten or more, you might begin to feel dizzy. Whenever you feel dizzy during your fast, you have to be careful standing up and sitting down too quickly. It happens because the body gets a little weak. There is no nourishment or anything, so naturally, the body feels uneasy. This doesn't mean you have to break the fast. Don't become negative or weak in your thinking. If you can still walk and do things, it shows you still have the strength to continue fasting.

During this time, your body heals and repairs itself. If sickness, cysts, infection, or cancer is growing in your body, it might begin to burn. You have to push a little bit if your body allows you. But if your body doesn't allow it, you will know it; you will not even be able to digest the water you are drinking. You will throw it up, and it serves as a warning. Your body is telling you not to go further without food. If your body cannot digest the lightest thing, water, it shows it is time to break the fast. It can be dangerous if you don't. Too much vomiting can cause the intestines to come up, and it can be life-threatening. In the "Breaking the Fast" section, I will detail the symptoms that indicate you need to break your fast and how to come out of the fast properly.

Feeling lethargic and weak

While fasting, you might feel foggy in the head and experience dizziness and weakness. This weakness will spread throughout your body, including the brain. Do the things you can do, but try to stay active, even if it is a little bit. For example, do a spiritual practice, chant mantras, walk, sit more instead of lying down, have some brain activity like putting together a puzzle, drawing, or writing. If you have no activity in this state, it can create trouble for you.

Feeling negative

It is natural to become negative while fasting. You are abstaining from the foods you enjoy. Cravings attack you. Your family might be telling you that it's not safe. Your body is aching and trying to adjust to the fast. These things can stir up emotions inside, so negativity attacks you. Suddenly you might get irritated. Even the smallest of things can trigger you. Why? Because you are on that level where the karma is on the surface, and little things can trigger the karma to come out. I have seen many monks in India that go through extreme anger those days they fast. Afterward, the anger fades. But that's what happens.

You are inviting this karma; negativity, anger, frustration, irritation, annoyance, and things like these to come up. This is the reason I always suggest seeking a positive environment. Even if these negativities attack you, being with positive people around you might offset how you react to them. It will help you not to get triggered much. But in the real sense, it is a good thing these emotions come to the surface. You don't have to create an enemy or enmity with the people around you. That's why, if you are in a positive environment, those around you will encourage you to walk, talk, do activities, and you will achieve success in your mission to fast.

Overall physical pain

It is quite normal to feel some pain and discomfort throughout the body. This is normal because the muscles and organs react to the fast since you are not feeding them, but this pain typically disappears in one or two days.

If the pain extends longer, this could happen due to your body constitution. You can refer to the "Recognizing your Body Type" section. Remember, if you do not clear your stomach before starting the fast, it will create much gastric trouble. When the food sits in your stomach, it creates gas. Eventually, this gas attacks your head and senses. You may get a terrible headache, and it can create a very uncomfortable feeling in the head; you cannot settle at all, you can't be peaceful, and you feel as if you are not in reality. That's why I strongly recommend preparing for extended fasting for at least two days in advance. It will help you clear your stomach ahead of time. Eat just liquids and let everything else in your stomach clear. And not only will your fast go more smoothly, but you will experience more healing.

Pain in a specific area

Other types of pain may surface during a fast. If the pain you experience is amplified in one area or part of your body, suppose the lower back, it means you already have trouble in the lower back. So, the fast will stir it up. It will bring more pain to the surface. Maybe an infection is growing in the lower back, and if the pain is too intense or persists too long, it's best to break the fast and see a doctor to get it checked. Maybe you need antibiotics. Small infections can be cleared by the fast, but not a significant infection that has been in the body for too long. If this is the case, I will not suggest fasting to take care of it.

If a person has a stomach or peptic ulcer, the fast will create a lot of trouble. The microbiome typically feeds off the foods people eat, but in fasting, they have nothing to eat, so if you have an ulcer, they can eat the stomach lining around the sore, making the ulcer bigger and creating more trouble. Anyone with stomach infections or ulcer-type conditions is best if they take care of it through medical, antibiotic, or naturopathic treatment before considering fasting. People with ulcers typically cannot eat spicy, acidic, or heavily spiced foods. Usually, the only spice the stomach can tolerate is turmeric. Any other spice will worsen the ulcer.

Small infections can be healed by fasting. The pain will be there, but it will last only one or two days. If the pain continues, then it indicates there could be a bigger problem, and I suggest you break the fast. Interpret small pain as healing and intense pain as a red flag into something bigger, which requires you to break the fast and see a doctor.

Sometimes old injuries that did not heal fully will surface too. The fast will try to heal and repair any leftover damage, but again if the pain becomes too intense, break the fast and visit your doctor. If not too severe, push through it and see if the fast can take care of it.

Blood pressure & shortness of breath

When fasting, you will experience lower blood pressure. The pressure calms down, but it also depends on how much pressure the person has. If a person suffers from high blood pressure, it is best not to do extended fasting. If anyone experiences shortness of breath, this could mean they have an underlying health condition or some health problems. Naturally, fasting does not create shortness of breath. Fasting can produce palpitations in the heart, but this does not mean it will increase blood pressure. However, if you dry fast, it will increase your blood pressure because there is no water in the blood. This is another reason not to dry fast for too long. One or two days is okay.

Vomiting

If your body has too much acid and you fast, automatically, the acid will want to come out. Here, I do not recommend extended fasting. You can fast for up to four days. After four days, if you continue to throw up more and more, you can get dehydrated and damage your intestines, stomach, and esophagus. Throwing up in excess clearly indicates your body is not ready for more prolonged fasting. If you have not vomited but feel continuously nauseous, it could also indicated that your stomach is not clear. Break the fast immediately if you experience this.

Emotions, feelings, and thoughts

Emotions go up and down during fasting. It is expected because people are not used to voluntarily tolerating the physical, emotional, and mental pain that comes with it. People can endure pain with sickness or illness because they have no choice. But emotions are dormant everywhere in the body, so when you stop eating, the body goes into shock, triggering and surfacing them while creating a lot of chaos inside.

Your feelings can go very high or very low. Likewise, thoughts can be very high and also very low. But it is up to you. Sometimes, though, to go high, you must go down first. Something important to know is that you should try not to break the fast when feeling low. It is not a good time. Wait for the flow to reverse. Break the fast when you feel high and full of energy. You may have to be patient for that moment to come, but it will be worth it. That is why the best tapa is patience. If you have patience, the flow will reverse, and all the emotions taking you downward will suddenly take you high again. When this happens, your feelings become clearer, and you feel a lot better. This process makes you stronger. Emotions will not affect you, whether you eat or not, or whether someone eats in front of you or not. This flow of emotions doesn't always reverse in one day. Sometimes it takes little time. Just be patient.

Feelings are like those of Prasanna Chandra Rajarshi. In the ancient Uttaradhyayana scriptures, you find the last spoken lecture by Tirthankara Mahavira. In this lecture, he shared the story of Prasanna

Chandra, who was a king and had renounced his kingdom to become a monk. One day while he was fasting, he was meditating in a standing pose. During that time, a minister passed through the area where he was meditating and uttered, "Look at you, you renounced your kingdom and left it to a teenager, your son. A king has attacked your kingdom, and now your son's life and kingdom are at stake! Shame on you for standing here!" This profoundly triggered him. While he was standing in a meditative state, all his emotions and attachment to his son suddenly came up, and he thought, "Who has the nerve to kill my son? I'm going to go there and kill them all!".

At the exact time, a king was visiting Tirthankara Mahavira. His name was King Shrenik. He asked, "My Lord, on my way here, I saw Prasanna Chandra Rajarshi, and he was standing in a meditative state. Can you tell me if he were to die right now, where his soul would go?" Tirthankara Mahavira responded, "He will go to the seventh hell." In shock, Shrenik replied, "What?!" And then the Tirthankara explained that whatever was said to him, he could not tolerate or digest. A few minutes later, Shrenik asked again, "What about now? If he dies, where would he go? Is he still there?" With the most surprising answer, Tirthankara Mahavira said, "Yes, he's still there, and he already got enlightened." Shrenik could not believe it and asked how this was possible. Tirthankara Mahavira explained that whoever said those things to him had helped him. His emotions got triggered too much. When the minister said the comment to him and was full of emotions, he went there to the battlefield mentally and got engrossed in killing the enemy soldiers. This was when Shrenik asked the first time. After, Prasanna Chandra exhausted his weapons. He grabbed his crown to use as a last resort. When he reached the crown, he touched his head and realized that he was bald and said, "I am a monk. What am I doing? Whose son, is he? Whose kingdom, is it?" So, he went higher and higher in his thoughts until he reached enlightenment. This was when Shrenik asked the second time.

Prassana Chandra only had *halu karma* left, which means "light karma." This incident helped him to go deep into his soul. The minister perhaps had animosity towards him, which explained why he said those things but look at how he became an important help on Prassana's path? Tirthankara Mahavira finally said, "Do you see all those angels? They are not coming to me. They are there to celebrate Prassana Chandra's enlightenment."

Unexpectedly, someone may help you too. Emotions can come out, and it can be a big help, like the incident that triggered Prasanna Chandra's emotions. Emotions touch rock bottom, and now they have nowhere to go other than up because they have touched the deepest part. This can happen in anybody's case. Emotions will go fully down, and that is a good sign. Just be patient and wait for it to reverse. It will allow you to burn significant karma quickly.

Time

Time always moves slower during fasting, that is for sure. Fasting is not always easy or comfortable. Any time there is an uncomfortable feeling, it feels like time doesn't move quickly enough. When people are happy, time passes so quickly. When they are not happy, become negative, or feel sick, they feel uneasy and uncomfortable, so time moves very slowly - sometimes, one hour feels like five hours. But it has nothing to do with time. It is how the person feels. That's why they say that hundreds of thousands of years pass so quickly in heaven because there is no suffering there. But in hell, it is the opposite. Time doesn't seem to pass because there is so much more suffering. Even here on this planet, if a person is tormented by sickness and pain, it won't be easy to go past even one night. Negative feelings or emotions slow time down.

The mind and willpower

The problem with the mind is that it is addicted to food. I've mentioned to you already that the biggest addiction is food. Therefore, the mind will not give up. It will play games on people. It will seduce and entice them with the best foods through dreams and thoughts. People become weak and negative because their mind is addicted to food, and they cannot break the addiction. It is challenging, so they eventually give up. Only people with strong willpower will complete their fast. People need to have a strong will. Everyone has a will, but maybe not strong. After fasting, the result is very satisfying. The more fasting you do, the more your willpower increases.

Sleeping

If you are fasting for just a few days, you should not experience sleep issues unless you already have insomnia. However, in a prolonged fast, you have to remember that your body is getting full rest. When the body gets to this level of rest, it doesn't need much more rest, especially if the person doesn't stay very active throughout the day. This is why many people can't sleep much, nor can they sleep continuously for a long time.

In addition, sleep happens because we put food in our bodies. Food is energy, and this energy creates warmness. When this warmness goes in the body, and food is being digested, it makes people sleep. But when you do an extended water fast, no energy or warmth is going in, so there is no real heat generating as it would when you eat food. The longer you fast, the more you stay awake. And the more you try to fall asleep, the more you stay awake too. It is best to understand that you will not sleep like you normally would when fasting for an extended time. Typically, when people stay up all night, they usually fall asleep early morning around three or four, and they might sleep for four to five hours, which is enough. If anyone's sleep gets altered, they have to change their thinking about sleeping at night only. I suggest for them to stay active more during the day. Read spiritual books, listen to a spiritual lecture or podcast, walk, meditate, write, work on your computer, and do spiritual practices. Occupy your mind, and time will pass quicker. At night you will find yourself not having trouble falling asleep. Don't rest or sleep too much during the day. This way, you have better chances of sleeping at night.

If people feel fatigued during the day, I do suggest taking short naps. Sometimes naps are enough; one hour here and there might be sufficient. But generally speaking, sleeping at night doesn't happen because there is no food in the stomach and because the body is too rested. Food and being tired are what make you fall asleep. Poor people don't have rich foods, but even if they eat a small piece of bread, it creates warmness in their bodies, and they can sleep at night.

Smooth fasting

When fasting goes smoothly, it means you cleared your stomach, the weather conditions were in your favor, you kept moving, and you stayed busy working on something. If anyone is trying to do an extended water fast, I suggest to continue working or being active for eight days. It will help have a more pleasant extended fast. Remember, after the eighth day and closer to the tenth, the body gets a little weak. One might feel dizzy standing and sitting down or might see black spots. If you feel weak but are still digesting the water and not experiencing pain, you are okay to continue fasting. That weakness doesn't mean you have a problem. It means your body is not receiving the nourishment, as I had explained before. This means your fast is going smoothly, and now you have the potential to heal many things in your body. Infection, harmful bacteria, and cancerous cells will burn. Many favorable results can happen. If weakness is your only symptom, keep pushing, and stay busy. Sitting idle will only make your thoughts about food, cravings, and breaking the fast get stronger. Don't give in. Time will come when the mind will surrender and accept that you are fasting for an extended period. Even if people eat in front of you, you will not get affected. Allow your smooth fast to help you heal your body and burn your karma.

Menstrual period

Many women wonder if they can fast while on their menstrual cycle. Yes, it doesn't affect anything. The period is a natural cleansing cycle anyway. If it's there, it's there, and it's not in your control unless you are taking hormones in the form of birth control. If it happens during your fast, it will help you burn even more karma because you might already feel uncomfortable, and on top of it, you are fasting, so it becomes a double benefit.

Some women may experience a cycle while fasting when it was not their time of the month or may experience spotting, especially when dry fasting. This happens because dry fasting creates a lot of heat, and heat can create a menstrual period. Sometimes women get their periods early because the fast will invite it as part of the cleanse. Not only are they purging and flushing toxins everywhere, but also, it will cleanse their body that way too. It will also help flush out excess iron as part of the cleanse. There is no resistance in the body; it happens naturally.

Negativity from others

Many people lack understanding and knowledge about fasting. They are not familiar with the concept that you can survive without food. They think you need food for survival. Naturally, they will feel concerned and will fear that something may happen to you. Undoubtedly, this can affect you. Those people will create some negativity inside of you. This is one reason people come to Siddhayatan to fast because they don't want to hear all the time, "It's not safe, you're going to die, one day is enough, this can't be good for you, etc." Eventually, when someone keeps hearing this over and over again, they quit, and they cannot last longer, even if they have the ability to do so. Sometimes it's helpful to avoid letting others know that you are fasting. You can let one person you trust. But for others, you can say you are enjoying a retreat. This way, you stay away from the negativity. Otherwise, you will be absorbing it, and the fast will not give you much of a positive benefit because you will be worried and negative most of the time.

In extended fasting, people do not have strong stamina because the body gets weaker. As a result, as I have mentioned, it is normal for anger, irritation, frustration, and negativity to come out during this time. In many people's cases, negativities surface in abundance. They criticize and judge others too much. They become totally negative. They'll look for little things to get mad at and blow them up way out of proportion. It can happen. It doesn't mean they are bad or negative people. It is just a reflection of the negativity surfacing. Imagine if you are fasting with eight other people, and everyone becomes negative at the same time. That negativity will become very strong. Collectively they will criticize everything. Even if loving, compassionate, and supportive people are around them, they will be hostile towards them. They will talk negatively the whole time they sit together, creating negative energy around other people too.

This is why it is so imperative to surround yourself with positive people from the very beginning. Don't get sucked into other people's negativities. Your good attitude, pure intention, and supportive environment can positively affect your fasting experience.

Nasal drainage, saliva, burping, and hiccups

Some people may experience an unusual amount of nasal drainage, saliva, burping, or hiccups. The excessive clear nasal discharge could result from too much mucus or kapha combined with excess retained water, which drains during the fast. Excessive burping and hiccups could result from too much gas or air in the body, and it releases during the fast.

The hyperproduction of saliva reflects that the person may consume foods that absorb too much water, such as rice. Rice grows in water. Therefore, people who consume too much rice might experience a disproportional amount of saliva generated during the fast. If these symptoms happen for one or two days, you should not get alarmed. However, if they persist and create too much discomfort, it is better to end the fast. Work on your diet and body. Try to balance the doshas as I explained in the "Recognizing your Body Type" section and improve your body's condition so you can fast longer with no issues.

Urine and bowel movements

The color of urine will change with water consumption. Water dilutes the pigments of yellows found in urine. When heavy toxins are coming out, the color of urine typically becomes darker, like amber color. But if the color becomes lighter, it doesn't mean you are not burning toxins. No matter what color, you will continue to cleanse your body and burn toxins. If the color is darker than usual or a different color, I recommend visiting your doctor as this could indicate underlying issues with your liver or something else.

Men with prostate gland enlargement issues will benefit from a fast. This problem happens in older age men between the ages of 50 and 60, and it can create many urination issues. Fasting will help to clear some of those issues affecting the bladder, liver, and urinary tract.

From the moment you swallow food, it can take up to five days for it to be fully digested and ready to leave your body. This all depends on each individual and the foods they eat. Food that sits in the intestines during a fast can create troubling gas, which can travel to the rest of the body. This gas can create severe headaches and pain in your body. As previously mentioned, it's important to clear your stomach before the fast. This is why I recommend eating more liquid foods at least two days before an extended fast. It will allow your stomach to clear. Otherwise, it can create gastric trouble.

For an extended fast, if you have a healthy digestive system, expect to have bowel movements within the first few days of the fast, but not after that. After the initial few days, you should not expect to have any bowel movements until after you break the fast. The fast will help clear your digestive system, improve your metabolism, reduce inflammation, and balance your microbiome. These natural healing processes get stimulated, so naturally, your overall health will improve.

What spiritual practices can be done while fasting?

Spiritual practices are many and practices like meditation are also considered a tapa, a fire. If somebody can enter a deep meditative state, they can burn mountain-high karma, and if they are fasting at the same time, it will burn very rapidly.

Here is a list of practices you can consider doing while fasting:

- Silence
- Mantra chanting/repetition
- Hatha Yoga
- Purnam Yoga
- Meditation
- Reading spiritual scriptures
- Pranayama
- Tratka
- Seva (selfless service)

Doing these practices will help you even more during the fast, but it will all depend on how you handle the practices. Practices keep you positive and active, and they also help you burn more toxins and burn your karma. I gave you an example earlier about reading scriptures; suddenly, what you read can hit you deeply. The result is that you can swiftly burn a lot of karma.

Silence is another tapa, but silence alone doesn't burn karma. Silence with knowledge burns karma. Silence requires a lot of discipline, and that discipline burns karma. When in silence, you are not only silencing your speech, you silence your thoughts, inner violence, negative emotions, and negative actions.

This is why it is important to engage in other spiritual practices while you fast, because even little things count and can make a big difference. Remember to do the practices with knowledge and wholeheartedly. Your fast will be more effective because combined with other practices, it will create a bigger fire. It is like adding ghee to the fire; the fire becomes shinier and more powerful, and it burns all the karma – ignorance, darkness, illusion, and negativities.

When is the best time to do pranayama while fasting?

Pranayama and Purnam Yoga is always more effective in the morning or evening. In the morning, trees release the most oxygen, so you can absorb it more to purify your body. When you do it in the evening, it helps you get a little more tired to sleep better at night. If you cannot do it early morning or in the evenings, don't let that stop you. Do your practice any time your schedule allows. In the bigger scope of things, doing this or other practices, will help accelerate burning karma.

What is Purnam Yoga?

Purnam Yoga is a system I realized while sitting on top of the Himalayas when I was doing intensive sadhana about 150 years ago, in a past life. Purnam Yoga is a unique system that combines specific movement with intensive breathing. I teach these techniques at Siddhayatan through various workshops, and people worldwide come to learn it. Purnam Yoga is used more for health purposes, because it helps to eliminate sickness in the body. Purnam means "perfect." It is perfect because it is very effective at cleansing the body.

The human body is the best and only instrument to grow spiritually; however, many things block it from being the healthiest body. These blockages can be removed through Purnam Yoga, and once removed, you can blossom through your instrument. If you're not healthy, then there is no connection between your body and spirituality. A sick body cannot follow spirituality much. In this aspect, Purnam Yoga is for health and spirituality, because it will create that kind of energy in your body that will help you advance on your spiritual path. Your aura will become much brighter, too. Purnam Yoga and fasting are an excellent combination to purge out all the toxins in your body. They create a tremendous wind to blow all the toxins, tension, stress, sickness, and negativities from your body.

What is Tratka?

Tratka is an ancient yogic and meditation technique I teach at

Siddhayatan, which brings out a lot of good qualities in you. In Tratka, you stare at a black dot without closing your eyes. As a result, your thoughts flow in one direction, and when they flow in one direction, they have a lot of power. If your thoughts flow in one direction and they are pure, they can help everyone around you. Your thoughts will no longer be scattered. It is like the sun rays. If trillions of rays are scattered, they have no power. But if you collect even 50 sun rays through a magnifying lens and they flow in one direction, they can create a fire. In a similar way, with Tratka, you create a fire that burns karma.

To practice Tratka, you will need a white sheet of computer paper, a U.S. quarter coin or a round object with the equivalent size, a pen, and a black marker. In the center of the sheet set the coin, with the pen, go around the coin to draw a circle. Last, use the black marker or black pen to fill in the circle. Tape the paper to the wall ensuring the black dot is at your eye level. To do the exercise, you can stand, sit on the floor cross-legged, or sit on a chair. You will need to be between two to three feet away from the wall. Adjust the distance according to what feels right for you. Once you adjust the distance, you will now stare at the black dot without blinking.

The first time you try it, you might blink within just a few seconds. Slowly build the tolerance to increase the time. Tears will roll down your eyes. It will feel uncomfortable with a burning sensation. This is normal, let the tension release the tears. When you stare, all the consciousness comes to your eyes and tremendous focused power can happen. All thoughts in your mind will stop. The eyes are very sensitive and delicate, and when all the consciousness comes into your eyes and there is no movement, the mind does not resist in this state. Thoughts disappear. It is an amazing state of being. It is the first step towards meditation. When you can do this without movement, meditation can happen.

Repeat Tratka two to three minutes at a time while sitting for thirty minutes each day, for at least forty-one days. After one year, you might be able to hold your stare for one hour. Do not allow moving air into the room; air conditioning, an open window, or a fan can hurt your eyes. If you have glaucoma or another eye condition, do not try doing Tratka for more than one or two minutes.

While fasting, one hour of Tratka with a pure intention, will burn a lot of karma, but it all depends on your intensity. A pure intention is when you do it because you wish to burn the negativities that surround your soul – your karma. If you are not fully there with pure intensity, it will not give you the highest result. To put things into perspective, it is possible to burn one hundred layers of karma while doing one hour of Tratka with the right intensity and purity.

Should salt or supplements be taken while fasting?

To experience real water fasting, you add nothing else to the water and do not take supplements. Once you add minerals, nutrients, or anything else, it becomes a partial fast. Partial fast means partial benefits. If you do it, you will still experience some benefits because you are not consuming solids. It is still considered better than a fast that entails taking food and solids, such as fasting during the Hindu celebration of Navaratri. But it will not give the results of a pure water fast.

In Navaratri, people fast for nine days by consuming lighter foods such as fruits, vegetables, juice, and milk. They are in a devotional and spiritual mood as they celebrate and honor Lord Rama and Goddess Durga. That joyful mood keeps them going for nine days. For them, that's beneficial because it is a spiritual celebration, and they are only eating light foods. Light foods give their system a little break. It doesn't have to work as hard. The intestines do not require much effort to break down that food. However, it will not reach the level needed to burn deep karma. Sometimes, even this type of fast can be very difficult, and if so, they can invite karma too.

Suppose a person is adding Himalayan salt, magnesium, lemon, or taking mineral water while wholeheartedly fasting. And they are in a positive and spiritual mood. There, they get more benefits than those doing the Navaratri fast. In that sense, this fast will be more effective at burning karma. It is up to how much benefit you wish to receive from the fast.

Some people think that by adding salt and minerals, they will be able to complete a 30-day water fast, but they don't realize that by not adding anything, they could get the same result physically in even ten days of pure water fasting. Yes, the minerals will nourish the person, and that is why they can hold the fast longer, but why go that long when you can reduce the time and still get the same benefit?

What should hygiene be like?

In the past, people did not do much to maintain good hygiene. Can you imagine how much they would smell? Their body odor was not good. They did not shower or anything, so their entire body was full of toxins on the surface.

Every pore takes out toxins, and toxins have a very bad smell. If there was no skin attached to the body, can you imagine what it would smell like? Nowadays, people who fast shower and take care of their bodies because they are typically fasting one day here and there. During extended fasting, some people choose not to shower or brush their teeth. Some people may do it to shut down their senses, as I did during my long fast. For this purpose, it is not a terrible thing if you are fasting by yourself. But if you are around others, it is best to take showers, brush your teeth, and keep good hygiene. A person fasting intensively is purging toxins continuously, and others can get affected by it. When you clean yourself, you feel fresher, which can help you maintain a good attitude during the fast.

In long-term fasting, some people's tongue will turn really white. This means a lot of bacteria and toxins are coming out through the tongue. You will see this happen more when people have too many toxins in the stomach. The tongue feels heavy and thick, and this makes people feel very uncomfortable. If you experience this, rinse and clean your tongue with hot water and a tongue scraper. The more you keep it clean, the better you will feel, and the less your tongue will smell. You can clean it two or three times per day to maintain good oral hygiene.

Remember that the senses are holes in your body, and when you fast, toxins will be expelled through your nose, teeth, tongue, skin, eyes, pores, and ears. Don't be too extreme or orthodox when doing extended fasting. Some people think by using toothpaste, you risk eating it and breaking the fast. I suggest to clean yourself, and you will feel better. Typically, people don't swallow the toothpaste; it just cleans the teeth and mouth. Rinse it well, and it should not affect you. Do not use salty water to clean your mouth; you might run a bigger risk of swallowing it, in this case.

What should be avoided while fasting?

In general, there are a few things I recommend that you do not do while fasting. I suggest not doing heavy physical labor, practicing strenuous exercise, smoking, engaging in intercourse, doing drugs, or taking medication.

Physical activity

Arduous physical work, exercise, or activity can deplete your organs and muscles. During the first eight days of an extended fast, you can do intensive spiritual practices such as yoga postures, pranayama, and Purnam Yoga, but after that, intensive sadhana should be avoided. There are some exceptional cases of people who have the energy to continue practicing intensive sadhana. However, too much can dry up your system and can hurt your organs and muscles. It's not beneficial during the fast and will be counterproductive to your healing. You can do these practices lightly throughout an extended fast.

There are other lighter activities you can consider doing like chess games, puzzles, or pastimes to keep your brain active. They will keep your mind occupied. You want to ensure your brain stays active but, most importantly, uplift your being by engaging in spiritual talks, thinking very high, activating your higher consciousness, sitting in the sun, reading, walking, journaling, creating art, or poetry. This is what people are supposed to do, purifying themselves, not only mentally and physically, but also spiritually. Find the right place where you can do these things. They will make your experience smoother and will help you burn your karma too.

Smoking

If you are a smoker, it will be quite difficult to stop smoking right away while fasting. If you can, avoid smoking while fasting. If you are doing an extended fast, you can ease into dropping smoking or vaping. Obviously, smoking defeats the purpose of the cleanse as you are inhaling more toxins. Those toxins can create trouble and even make you sick while fasting. That's why it is best to drop smoking before you begin fasting.

Being around others

While fasting, you are purging toxins out. Those toxins that your body releases can affect others, especially if they stay close to you unless they are in the same boat and fasting too. This level of effect happens only when you are doing an extended fast. Up to one week of fasting will not affect much. However, even after three to four days of fasting, I suggest not getting too close to others. Why? They could be sensitive to the toxins you are releasing, and they can get sick from you. While the person fasting purifies their bodies and expels toxins, others could collect those toxins by inhaling or coming in close contact with them. That is why I also suggest keeping good hygiene.

Negativities

Avoid people, situations, or places which can aggravate, worry, or negatively affect you. Stay around people and in an environment supportive of your fasting goals.

Intercourse

Understand that all organs get weak during a prolonged fast, and the reproductive organs are no exception. In an extended water fast, they get weak when the healing process begins. I suggest to married couples to sleep separately if one of them is fasting. Many people are unaware of this and they make the mistake by engaging in sexual intercourse. Fasting is a healing process; therefore, stay alone in your room to avoid this situation. I suggest not having intercourse at all because this will create a lot of trouble for you. Your organs are weak. While fasting, you are supposed to be fully celibate those days. You are purifying yourself totally. You are not only purifying your body or mind; you are purifying yourself spiritually. Spiritual purification means you stay away from temptations, pleasure, desires, and anything that stimulates your senses. You shut all your senses. Lift yourself up. By purifying yourself in this way, you will burn a lot of karma.

Medicine and drugs

In long-term water fasting, I do not recommend taking medication. In short fasts, between two to four days maximum, you can take the necessary medications that do not require food. Medication can hurt your body while fasting, so avoid it. Dropping medicine abruptly can be dangerous and can adversely hurt you, so consult with your doctor to stop taking them safely before you fast.

Some people explore or consider taking drugs in the name of spirituality or healing, but I never recommend taking any drug or substance which alters your natural state, even if they believe it to be natural or spiritual. Drugs and medication are toxins. Drugs like psychedelics or ayahuasca make you hallucinate and not see the reality. This is not healing nor spiritual. In very rare and exceptional cases, healing might occur, but it is so rare that I do not recommend it. Heal yourself naturally through the water fast. It is a safer route. Drugs can make you go crazy, and I have seen it happen too often.

CHAPTER 13

BREAKING THE FAST

It is quite normal to feel irritated, uncomfortable, tired, and a little weak, but it is not usual to feel unwell. You need to listen to your body and break the fast any time you feel uncertain about your well-being or simply any time you feel ready to break it. I have said several times it is best not to force fasting. When your body gives you too much trouble, it is an immediate sign you need to stop fasting. Remember, breaking the fast early doesn't mean you are weak. It shows you have the strength and wisdom to listen to your body. But if you are not forcing the fast and wish to complete a long water fast, it is vital to know a few symptoms that may indicate that it is time to break the fast.

The first symptom to be wary of is if you feel like you are getting too weak. Your legs, arms, abdomen, muscles, and bones all feel weak. The weakness I am referring to is when you cannot even move. Your body becomes so debilitated that you cannot stand or walk. This is your body telling you to do something – to break the fast.

The second symptom to be aware of is if you faint or feel continuously dizzy. During fasting, it is normal to feel dizzy when you stand or sit, but if you feel it all the time and it gets to the point of fainting, it is time to break the fast. Your body is telling you that you cannot proceed further into the fast.

The third symptom to recognize is if you can no longer digest the water you are drinking. How do you know if you are not digesting water? You cannot keep it down, and you regurgitate it. There is a distinction when vomiting happens early in the fast – if it happens early on, it means there's too much acid in the body. Let the acid come out and see if you feel better. But the regurgitation I am referring to happens when you do an extended fast, and you have reached the limit your body can handle, indicating it is time to stop fasting. Even if you throw up once, I suggest you end the fast.

When I fasted for 32 days, I experienced severe pain but never vomiting. Vomiting during fasting can be very dangerous. If your goal was 30 days and at day 15 you throw up, you need to end the fast right away. If you do not break the fast and the vomiting continues, it can become so intense that it can bring the feces out of your intestines, and it can spread throughout the body – this can hurt your body and become fatal. Be aware that if vomiting is too frequent at any time during your fast, it can also damage your esophagus due to the acid. Forceful or extreme vomiting can create tears in the esophagus' inner lining and create more problems for you. Don't risk it at all. Break the fast; otherwise, you can lose your precious body.

What are reasons to break an extended fast early?

The body comprises hundreds of trillions of microbes, and trillions of them reside in your digestive system, especially in the large intestine. These microbes are bacteria, viruses, fungi, and parasites. Collectively, with their genetic material, the microbiota in your body is called the microbiome, and they may weigh as much as five pounds of your body. What is important to note here is that the microbiome is essential for human life, development, immunity, and nutrition. The gut microbiome also directly affects the brain, nervous system, and mental health.

Fasting is very effective at restoring your gut microbiome composition; it strengthens and generates good bacteria's growth while eliminating the harmful ones. People who fast regularly will have a healthier digestive system. However, fasting longer than what your body needs can kill even the good microbes essential for survival. That is why, during fasting, it is imperative to maintain the five pounds of microbes needed to be alive. Otherwise, you will jeopardize your health. Scientifically and generally, the human body can survive for 90 days drinking water only, but it is not for everyone. Fat can burn during the fast, but that is why we keep drinking water. Minerals in the water help maintain healthy microbiome levels to a certain point. But water is not enough. This is why you cannot dry fast for too long. Dry fasting can disrupt and destroy the appropriate microbiome levels very quickly.

Besides microbes, human cells also benefit from fasting. It is essential to understand that cells get damaged due to oxygen deficiencies, toxins, and lack of nutrients. When too much damage is done, the organs and tissues can fail. During fasting, cells can repair and regenerate themselves through a process called autophagy, which allows the cells to destroy and recycle those damaged parts to rebuild new and healthy cells. This process is vital for disease prevention, good health, and longevity. But if you fast beyond your body's limit it can also affect the cells.

In the long term, both human cells and microbes need food for vital nutrients to generate energy, stay alive, and be healthy. When the body has had enough fasting or when the body reaches the point where there is no fat or waste materials to eat from, the cells can turn to protein or muscle tissue to create energy. This process can weaken the organs and muscles, and you can compromise your health. At this point, the person will feel it. They will feel uncomfortable as if they were dying. They will feel very unsettled and not themselves.

Remember that any time during a fast, if you find yourself very weak, not digesting water, and becoming dizzy to the point of fainting, you need to break the fast. If a person is stubborn to break it, they can lose their body. Certain bodies cannot last long while fasting. These bodies are not ready for prolonged fasting. Their karma does not allow them to, and if they force it, they can die. If any of these symptoms are present, break the fast. If there are no signs of them, then you can continue fasting.

What are the wrong ways to break the fast?

I consider breaking the fast equally important as the fast itself. Breaking the fast safely is very difficult. If you do not break it safely, you can damage your entire system, which gives you the opposite result of what you were trying to achieve during your fast. Sometimes it may appear that you have safely come out of the fast, but the negative or damaging effects don't appear until later. In extended fasting, out of excitement, cravings, or lack of knowledge, many people indulge in unhealthy foods or items that do not necessarily go well with the body's state after the fast. During fasting, the body is turned off, and you must gently turn it back on.

Before learning how to break your fast, it is essential to understand how not to break it. When you fast for a short period, one or two days, you can eat almost anything as it will not affect your body much. But even if it will not hurt your body much, I still suggest that you eat something light to break the fast with. In the Hindu tradition, they like to drink some juice in the beginning, but they are only fasting for one or two days. However, in extended fasting, I do not suggest breaking the fast with juice, fruits, or watermelon, as some people may indicate.

In extended fasting, the body is fully calmed down. If someone who has fasted for one month wants to break the fast with juice or fruits, they need to understand that certain juices or fruits like watermelon are cold in nature. When you eat something cold in nature, it will calm down your body even more rather than wake it up, and when breaking the fast, you want your system to be activated – it needs to be turned back on, not kept or put back to sleep.

The watermelon's nature can impair your system. There are always exceptions. Some people may not get affected by eating it, but it will hurt people's systems, in general. Those who crave it or have this idea to break the fast with watermelon will want to eat at least half of it or the entire watermelon on the first day. These people will get sick. But if they are stubborn and insist on breaking it with watermelon, I will suggest having only a few small pieces. A few pieces will not hurt in rare cases, but it will also not help wake up their system effectively. In extended fasting, I do not recommend breaking the fast with watermelon. This is why you have to break the fast gently and carefully.

When you fast, you have put forth so much effort to purify your body. Whether you have fasted for one or thirty days, I do not suggest breaking the fast with any meat products. Chicken broth or bone broth is very wrong. In prolonged fasting, meat products can especially hurt your system forever. I advise that no meat products enter your stomach. All meats are heavily toxified. Suppose a person is fasting for healing reasons and not necessarily for spiritual reasons; no matter the reason, it is still fasting. When they break the fast, they go to a restaurant and order fish or chicken soup. They will hurt themselves because their system is not ready for this level of heavy toxins. Meat is considered more toxic than vegetables, so it is wrong to break the fast with it. Healthy vegan and vegetarian foods are always the most suitable.

When breaking the fast after five days, I do not suggest eating raw items. After a reset of your microbiome, you do not want to risk ingesting harmful bacteria. The body is not yet fully turned back on. The body and immune system are weak, and if you consume harmful bacteria, such as E. coli or Salmonella, your body's response might not be strong enough to fight against them. You need to wake up your system slowly, and naturally, the immune system will get stronger if you break the fast the right way. Boiled, steamed, or cooked food will always be a safer option. Raw is the incorrect way to break the fast. Raw items include juices, fruits, or vegetables. After safely breaking the fast for three days, you can then eat raw items.

I encourage you always to eat boiled or cooked food. When cooked, it is less dangerous because the bacterias get killed. But if you eat raw vegetables, as raw-vegan people do, you are taking a risk. You might get affected by the foodborne diseases. There will always be exceptions. Some people may not get affected by it, but for the most part, eating raw foods puts your health at risk. What if the food is contaminated with bacteria, viruses, or parasites? These are microorganisms that are not visible. Even when our monks and nuns want to eat salad, we suggest adding some salt or lemon. Why? Because the salt and lemon will help eliminate the bacteria. Sometimes, even the lemon and salt will not work because certain microbes are tough to get rid of.

Suppose a person wants to eat a salad, and the salad has spinach. Sprouts and leafy green vegetables, like spinach, are the most linked to bacterial infections due to E. coli. Even if you wash them or purchase the triple-washed prepackaged greens, it is not guaranteed that it will eliminate these harmful bacteria. If you ingest it, it can make you sick, and you can end up in the hospital. This is why people in India always boil spinach. They have this knowledge, so they don't take the chance and don't eat it raw. I suggest to everyone to do the same. Don't risk your health.

Breaking the fast the wrong way is inviting all the trouble. It is like a bull standing in front of you, and let's say the bull is considered a disease, and somebody says, "Hey bull, come and hit me." He's going to hit you, no doubt. In prolonged fasting, breaking the wrong way can have detrimental consequences, and you will regret it for the rest of your life. When people break the fast, they crave a lot of highly processed fast food and fried foods. If people eat these foods, they can ruin their system, and it can take years or a lifetime for your body to pick up again. They have to be careful. If someone had so much discipline to fast for 30 days, why not have control for four more days during the refeeding process? This is why I say fasting is easy to do, and breaking the fast is more difficult. Why? Because hunger and cravings attack you, and if you do not have discipline, control, and knowledge, you will hurt your whole system. People binge without considering the consequences. But if you follow the advice shared here, you will be safe.

Here is a list of foods you DO NOT want to consume for breaking the fast:

- acidic foods
- spicy foods
- meats (beef, pork, poultry, fish, etc.)
- fried foods
- eggs
- candy or sweets
- bone broth
- raw foods (including raw fruits and vegetables)
- watermelon
- cold nature foods
- junk food
- sodas
- coffee
- alcohol

Why do "fasting experts" suggest breaking a fast with juice, fruits, or watermelon?

It may appear like these doctors or "experts" know what they are talking about at first sight. But writing a book does not mean they are truly experienced at fasting. Many have not even done an extended 30-day only-water-fast. So, when they write about fasting, it is like when doctors prescribe medication without having tried the medicine themselves. While they have never taken the medicine, they still recommend it because the Food and Drug Administration approves it, but they are not sure if it will work. They prescribe it, and if it doesn't work, they prescribe a different one. Consequently, making decisions based on what the system says to do and not based on their own lived experience. They go patient by patient, constantly experimenting to see what works with each one of them. In the same way, these "fasting experts" are just experimenting and advising without experience. But with fasting, it is never a one-size-fits-all process or solution.

If a doctor writes about fasting, that doesn't mean the book is authentic. People may think, "Well, it is written by a doctor. It must be true." Yes, maybe they have done the research, and perhaps they read other people's books, and during that research, they find out medically how the kidneys react when you don't drink water. Most doctors do not recommend fasting. They think you are depleting your body from all energy sources, so they are against it. And those doctors writing books about it have not gone through their own experience. So, whose knowledge should you listen to? Those who have gone through it themselves. Like I went through this experience so I can tell you about it. If I am a doctor or not, I know it. Why? Because I went through it by myself and I have personally guided thousands of people through it, and I can advise you on the right things to follow. I care about you and your spiritual growth and want to ensure you have the right guidance.

Why are certain foods craved during a fast?

Fasting brings up the taste of what people like to eat in their daily lives, so they will naturally crave them. People are addicted to certain foods, even healthy ones, so when they fast and suppress the cravings, they can get out of control when they break the fast. Notice how when people are not fasting, let's say they like papaya, and if papaya is not available when they go shopping, they don't really care too much about it. But if they are fasting, suddenly the craving for papaya will surface, and they go purchase one, and if it's not available, they feel horrible because they want it badly.

Whatever people like to eat in their lives, fasting will bring those tastes up on the surface, and they will crave it. Spiritual understanding during a fast helps you gain control of your senses. It is a discipline. And discipline is of utmost importance. In extended fasting, as mentioned, breaking the fast properly is the most difficult thing. It's not easy. Up to one week of fasting requires one day to refeed carefully. After one week, it is better to break it the right way. Otherwise, you are inviting the bull to hit you, and instead of getting better, you get sick.

How to safely break the fast?

Traditionally, the Samanic tradition follows a very safe system, which I recommend to follow. You can use this method after any fasting length. For extended fasts, such as 21-30 days, I strongly suggest you follow it. You can break the fast any time you are ready, but preferably, I recommend starting in the morning at least 48 minutes after sunrise. During the day, your digestive system is more active than at night, making it more effective at digesting the foods you will be reintroducing. At the end of this chapter, you will find the detailed recipes we use at Siddhayatan to help our guests break their fast. It will help you have a safe experience.

In the morning, for breakfast, the first item to consume is a cup of clove tea. Clove tea will gently wake up your system. Clove is an antiseptic with antimicrobial properties. It helps to kill harmful and infectious bacteria growing in the body. When you consume it after fasting, it helps to clear off any of these bad bacteria sitting in your small intestine and colon. In addition, clove creates a little heat, and it will not let bad bacteria be heavy on your body as it calms them down. You can add some organic or raw sugar to sweeten the tea if you do not have a sugar allergy. I suggest not to use honey. Honey, combined with clove, can create problems. Both clove and honey are hot in nature, and too much heat can create trouble. If you use organic or raw sugar, even a small amount will help your cells break it down into glucose to generate and bring back some energy.

Still at breakfast, following the clove tea, you drink a cup of special milk. If you are vegan or lactose intolerant, you can use a plant-based milk. In the milk, you mix almond paste and a small amount of ghee. The milk, almonds, and ghee reintroduce essential protein, vitamins, fat, fiber, and minerals to nourish the cells and the gut microbiome. The ghee also helps create lubrication in your whole system and makes the intestines soft to release dry stool stuck in them. In our Samanic tradition, it has always been known that ghee and the fiber in the almonds help eliminate waste material from the intestines. After you drink the tea and milk, do not consume any water for the next hour. I suggest that you lie down and rest after. Let your body turn on and absorb all the nutrients. Eat nothing else until lunchtime. If you did a dry fast, first drink water. You may be very thirsty, but don't drink the water too fast. After, give your system about 5 minutes to wake up and hydrate. Then you can continue with the clove tea and milk.

A few hours later, during lunchtime, you have a *Kala Chana* broth. Kala Chana are black chickpeas, and they offer an abundance of nutrients – from iron to protein. You let the beans boil for two to three hours until they are fully cooked. You will need to check on the beans as the water evaporates. Add water as needed. The body is not ready to digest the beans yet, so you will only take the broth, which will have all the nutrients released from the beans. You add some salt to the broth, and you can add some ghee. The broth will give you strength and added lubrication for your body. Like with the first two drinks, do not drink water during or one hour after consuming the broth. Eat nothing else until dinner time.

Usually, after the first two meals, you experience a bowel movement. If not, it means the body needs a little more lubrication. In the evening, for dinner, you will have a more liquid version of *Kitchari* – an easy-to-digest combination of mung beans, rice, ghee, and a little salt. This combination will continue to help you recover your strength and will help add more valuable nutrients. You can have water during and after this meal, but eat nothing else. This last meal will create more lubrication and will help you sleep well at night, especially if you have not slept well due to the fast.

If you did a short fast, you could eat regular light foods on the second day. But if you fasted for over seven days, proceed to the next regimen. The second day is safe to reintroduce fruits, but not too much, only a few pieces. For breakfast, you can have light oatmeal and some fruit. For lunch, have a vegetable soup with veggies chopped small, and as an option, add a tiny amount of rice and mung beans. For dinner, have a more solid version of Kitchari. On this second day, it is a good idea to add some lemon or lime juice to the fruit you eat, as well as to the soup. This will help disinfect the food you are eating and will prevent harmful bacteria from entering your body. As a tip, if you feel like you have too many toxins sitting on your tongue, you can have some lemon pickle. In India, people have a small piece of lemon pickle, and they suck it a little bit, and it helps to disinfect the mouth. You can find lemon pickle at the Indian market, and you will only need a tiny piece.

And this is the way you start, little by little reintroducing foods. For every week of fasting you completed, you need one full day of refeeding. On the third and fourth days, stick to oatmeal, soups, cooked vegetables, Kitchari, mung beans (daal), rice, and some fruits. After the second day, you might feel very thirsty, but be careful. Many people start drinking too much water, and too much water is not good. You still need other types of aliments to clear your stomach first. Once you have your first bowel movement, you switch to safe mode.

Be sure to only eat these meals. No snacks, drinks, or other foods between. Refeeding requires discipline. Watch your portions and try not to overeat. Otherwise, you will not feel well. If you maintain discipline during your refeeding, you will subsequently clear your stomach, and you can switch to regular foods with no issues at all and safely.

REFEEDING RECIPES

CLOVE TEA

Ingredients:

- 2 cups water
- 4 - 5 whole cloves
- 1/2 - 1 tsp organic sugar

Directions:

1. Break the cloves in half and boil them in the water until the water turns golden brown. If the water is too light or pale in color it means the cloves have not released enough flavor. If the color gets too dark, the flavor might be too strong.
2. Strain the water and serve yourself one cup of the tea. Add 1/2 to 1 teaspoon of sugar and enjoy.

Notes: This is the first item to break the fast with. Sip on it and drink it slowly. Start with one cup of tea only to leave room for your second drink. Ironically, you might feel full too quickly. Consume vegan sugar, free of bone char.

SPECIAL MILK

Ingredients:

- 1-1/2 cups of organic milk or plant-based milk
- 10 peeled almonds
- 1 tsp ghee
- 1 tsp organic sugar

Directions:

1. Overnight, soak the almonds in purified water. The next morning (the day of breaking fast), remove the dirty water and rinse the almonds in clean water. Next, peel off the skin.
2. Blend the 10 peeled almonds with the 1-1/2 cup of milk. If you do not have a blender, you can use a mortar and pestle to ground the almonds to create a paste.
3. In a small saucepan, pour the blended milk or the milk and almond paste. Over medium-low heat, then bring it to a boil. Lower the heat and keep on low heat for 2 minutes.
4. Add the 1/2 teaspoon of ghee and with a mixing spoon, mix the ghee until it integrates with milk.
5. Pour the milk in a cup, add the sugar, and enjoy.

Notes: Sip on it and drink it slowly. Use a spoon to stir it well. Start with one cup. If you still have room and do not feel too full, feel free to mix any leftover clove tea with any remaining milk you have and drink it. Do not drink any water for one hour after the tea and milk.

KALA CHANA BROTH

Ingredients:

- 1/2 cup of kala chana (black chickpeas)
- 4 cups of water
- 1/2 tsp Himalayan or sea salt
- 1/4 tsp turmeric powder
- 1/4 tsp coriander powder
- 1/4 tsp cumin powder
- 1/2 small tomato chopped
- 1/4 small onion finely chopped (if you're not Vaishnava or Jain)
- 1/2 tsp oil or ghee
- 1 tsp finely chopped cilantro
- 1/4 tsp ginger (optional)

Directions:

1. Overnight, soak the black chickpeas in clean water. The next morning drain the water and rinse the beans. Add the drained beans to a stockpot with the 4 cups of water and 1/2 teaspoon of salt. In medium-high heat, bring the water to a boil. Then reduce the heat to low and boil the beans for two hours or until fully cooked. Check the water level periodically. If the water evaporates too much, add water accordingly.

2. To season the broth, you will first sauté the chopped onion

on a separate pan until it turns light golden brown. Turn off the heat for now. From the stockpot, pull about two full cups of broth and pour into the same pan where the onion is.

3. Extract 10 - 15 black chickpeas and, with a fork, thoroughly mash them. Add them to the onion and broth mixture. Make sure the chickpeas are fully mashed; otherwise, you will have trouble digesting them.

4. Add the rest of the ingredients: tomato, turmeric, coriander, cumin powder, ginger (optional), ghee, and cilantro. If needed, add salt to taste. Turn the heat back on and bring to a boil over medium-high heat. Once it reaches boiling point, drop the temperature to low, cover, and let it cook for 10 minutes. Pour in a large bowl and enjoy.

Notes: Eat the broth slowly. Do not drink water while you are eating it and for one hour after that.

LIQUID KITCHARI

Ingredients:

- 2 tbsp split mung beans
- 2 tbsp basmati rice
- 3 cups water
- 1 tsp coriander powder
- 1/2 tsp turmeric powder
- 1/2 tsp chopped cilantro
- 1 tsp ghee

- Salt to taste

Directions:

1. Wash the basmati rice and mung beans thoroughly. After washing, place them in a medium saucepan with the 3 cups of water. In medium-high heat, bring the water to a boil.

2. Reduce the heat to low and add the rest of the ingredients: salt, turmeric, coriander, ghee, and cilantro.

3. Cook on low heat for about 15 minutes or until the beans and rice are fully cooked. Serve in a bowl and enjoy.

Notes: If you overcook the mung beans, they might dissolve in the water. You can serve yourself a second portion if you still feel hungry. You may drink some water along with this meal and thereafter.

What else is expected while breaking the fast?

If you follow the methods I have shared with you, you will feel better immediately. Your strength and energy will come back relatively quickly. Negativities will subdue, and you will feel light and happy. If you could not sleep well during the fast, you will sleep better soon after breaking. On the first or second day of breaking the fast, expect to have a bowel movement – if it happens on the first day, it shows you are having a very smooth transition.

PART V:

OPTIMAL LIVING

CHAPTER 14

LIVING YOUR BEST SPIRITUAL LIFE

After fasting, if you wish to continue to experience good health, joy, balance, spiritual growth, and happiness, you must make lifestyle changes. Spirituality is practicality, which means you must practice it, and guidance is necessary to optimize your life and potential. You must continue to purify your body, mind, speech, and soul. You need guidance, understanding, discipline, and much effort to realize and free yourself. Karma will not go anywhere unless you put the effort to dissolve it. Therefore, fasting is a valuable tool you can continue to use to rid yourself of darkness, pain, suffering, ignorance, and illusion – all karma.

Besides fasting, I advise you to follow a vegetarian diet post-fasting.

For spiritual reasons, it is the best and lightest diet to help you grow spiritually. As you now know, it is the first step of non-violence, and it can take you closer to experiencing oneness. Vegetarianism keeps your body light and healthy. I am not opposed to eating junk or fried foods sometimes, but try not to eat them regularly as they are considered heavy, toxic and addictive. It is best to avoid them, and if feasible, eat as fresh and natural as possible. If you eat a healthy vegetarian diet, you will experience longevity and optimal living. In addition, it prevents you from collecting more karma, which you are trying to dissolve. By respecting, loving, and caring for all living beings, you will expand yourself.

Add spiritual practices to this equation, and you will live a more balanced life. I encourage you to learn Purnam Yoga to help you purge more toxins and remove tension, stress, and trauma from your body. Meditation will help you connect deeply with your soul. Mantras create beautiful, protective, healing, and divine energy; chant or repeat mantras to generate this energy. Traditional yoga postures help to keep your body healthy and flexible. Learn more techniques through an enlightened master's guidance to help you achieve your ultimate goal of spiritual awakening and liberation.

In summary, here is a list of recommendations for optimal spiritual living:

- Continue fasting, based on my recommendations. Add it to your calendar to make it easier to remember.

- Follow a balanced, light, and healthy vegetarian diet.
- Learn about the nature of the foods you eat and learn how to combine them accordingly.
- Avoid consuming too much oil, sweets or sugar, salt, junk food, fried and processed foods.
- Work on not collecting more karma and dissolving the karma you already have.
- Practice Purnam Yoga and traditional yoga postures.
- Meditate at least 5 minutes each day.
- Repeat mantras daily.
- Use your skills, talents, time, and resources to practice Seva - selfless service.
- Keep a pure intention always.
- Eradicate the violence in your thoughts, speech, and actions.
- Always seek right guidance to ensure you are going in the right direction.
- Read spiritual books that will help you gain an understanding about yourself and the spiritual path.
- Keep your body pure. Avoid smoking, taking drugs, drinking alcohol, and eating meats, including eggs.
- Try to live a life free of stress and worries.
- Be content with yourself and your life.
- Forgive and don't hold grudges and resentment.
- Gain mastery over your senses and mind.
- Real change begins with you, so look for ways to make yourself better each day.
- Don't judge others. Inside each person, there is an

entire universe. Every person is different. It is best to focus on yourself.

    ♦   Life is too short, don't waste it being angry or negative. Do good things for yourself and others.

What mantras are recommended for spiritual growth?

I encourage everyone to learn and repeat the Namokar Mantra. The Namokar mantra is a universal mantra that anyone, regardless of creed or faith, can recite. It is a very beautiful mantra that recognizes and honors the most auspicious and divine beings in the universe. They represent all the qualities that one can strive to achieve with effort and when you recite it, you appreciate the laying groundwork these divine beings have set for the path of enlightenment and liberation. The person who understands the mantra's meaning and repeats it sincerely becomes pure, divine, and humble.

<u>Namokar Mantra</u>
Namo Arihantaanam
Namo Siddhaanam
Namo Ayariyaanam
Namo Uvajjhaayaanam
Namo Loe Savva Saahunam
Eso Pancha Namokaaro
Savva Paavappanaasano
Mangalaanamcha Savvesim
Padhamam Havai Mangalam

The meaning of the mantra is:

I bow down to all Arihantas, enlightened masters who have won victory over themselves. I bow down to all Siddhas, liberated souls who have ended their karma. I bow down to all Acharyas, the spiritual masters or divine spiritual leaders. I bow down to all Upadhyayas, the divine spiritual teachers who teach about the spiritual path. I bow down to all Sadhus, the nuns and monks who have taken the 5 great vows: *Ahimsa* - non-violence, *Satya* - truthfulness, *Asteya* - non-stealing, *Brahmacharya* - celibacy, and *Aparigraha* - Non-possessions. This five-fold salutation destroys all sin, and among all auspicious things, this mantra is the most auspicious one.

CHAPTER 15

FINAL THOUGHTS & RECOMMENDATIONS

If people have a true mission to burn karma, I recommend they water fast for a total of 30 days in one year. This is the ideal number of days to burn karma, and it can be achieved by breaking it into single days or segments. I would not suggest doing a 30-day water fast every year, but I do suggest, however, that at least once in your lifetime, you experience a one-month fast only if your body allows you to. It will depend on your body type, but you can work on your body to make it happen. But in general, for those serious spiritual practitioners whose intention is to burn as much karma as possible, they should ideally fast for 30 days, in segments, throughout the year. This is the best, fastest, and safest way to do it. Be aware that you are inviting the karma to burn, it may not be pleasant, but for your soul, it is the best gift.

How often should people fast for the best health possible?

If you are fasting for spiritual reasons, you automatically get the health benefits. But to achieve good health through fasting, you must incorporate good habits, exercise, a proper vegan or vegetarian diet, and not add any more toxins to your body. Meats, tobacco, drugs, alcohol, and heavily processed foods are full of toxins, so it is counterproductive to have them if you are trying to purify your body.

To prevent cancer, I suggest fasting for at least 21 days a year. And just like I mentioned before, you can spread them throughout the year. You can do a water fast once or twice a month. Single fasts are considered 24 hours. And if you are on the right diet, a healthy and balanced vegan or vegetarian diet, cancer cells cannot grow in the body because your 21 days of fasting will help burn the cancer cells. That is the best calculation without doing anything else. And 21 days is not too much in one year. It is not continuous fasting, you can spread it out, and you will have a high chance of staying away from cancer. Don't wait until it is too late to take care of your body. For some people, the damage is irreversible, and no matter what they do, it doesn't work. Prevention is the cure to all diseases.

When are the best days to fast?

For spiritual purposes, I advise you to fast on a full or new moon. The new moon happens once a month when it aligns itself between the earth and the sun. Because the moon calendar is not synchronized with our calendar, there may be 13 new moons in one year. The new moon offers the darkest night of the month. During this time, there is not much energy. There is too much density in the darkness, and you need something to lift you up and inspire you to purify yourself. When you fast during the new moon, the darkness is beneficial to clear toxins you have accumulated in your body.

I highly recommend fasting during a full moon. A full moon happens two weeks after a new moon when the sun fully illuminates it. Since the body comprises 70% water, it gets affected by the moon's gravity pull. The full moon alters emotions, moods, and behaviors. It is often reported there is an increase in violence, criminal activities, fights, and breakups during this time. People don't know why the erratic behavior occurs, but it is because the moon affects our emotions. During holidays like Thanksgiving, it is best if there is no full moon. Otherwise, it will create a lot of trouble among families, and instead of enjoying their time together, they will fight. But if someone is in a spiritual environment or celebrating a spiritual holiday as they do in India, they will think about it spiritually. They will say, "Hey, it's a full moon. Let's fast so that it can help us discipline our emotions." And when you fast and are in higher thinking, your emotions naturally calm down, even if they are on the surface.

Consider using a new and full moon's timing to help you maximize your fast. Both can positively help you. During a full moon, fasting will calm down your emotions, which allows you to become more disciplined with your feelings – they will not be that strong to make you fight, make regretful decisions, commit a crime, or have volatile reactions. So, you never know, that's why it is always a good idea to surround yourself with a positive and spiritual atmosphere, and when you fast, your emotions will calm down. And during a new moon, the fast will help to lift you up from the darkness.

If you cannot fast throughout the year, I encourage you to consider fasting during the 8-day spiritual celebration of Paryushan. During the month of August or September, millions of people across India and the world focus on the inner world, and disengage from the senses. They live around their soul. It is a time of fasting and being still. Fasting can be done for one, eight, or thirty days, depending on how much a person can tolerate and wishes to purify their being. Paryushan is the only purely spiritual celebration where there is no indulgence through the senses. It is a time to feed the soul through fasting, spiritual lectures, sadhana, awareness, self-analysis, and forgiveness. When you fast during this time, you will be joining the millions of fasting people in a positive and spiritual mood. Collectively, you will create beautiful energy to help bring balance to our world.

What are your final thoughts about fasting?

As a final recommendation, I advise people to fast for spiritual upliftment rather than for physical reasons. As a spiritual practitioner, your goal is to grow spiritually. You fast to purify your soul and get rid of all karma – ignorance, illusion, darkness, and pain. Those who fast for spiritual growth reap the most benefits. All other physical and mental benefits become a byproduct of fasting. Fasting for spiritual growth allows you to heal, transform and liberate yourself.

People are mentally very weak. Even though it is scientifically known that the human body can survive without food for a maximum of 90 days, they have a very difficult time even fasting for one day. I am not an extremist and do not suggest fasting for 90 days, but I want to encourage you to fast for however long your body is ready to handle. If it lets you do four days, do four days. If eight days, do eight days. But if you cannot go further, don't force it and break the fast. Forcing fasting can make you lose your body, and we don't want that to happen. Look for all the symptoms I've shared with you. Listen to your body and follow my advice.

When anger and negativities surface, it is a good thing. But be careful. If you are around others, sometimes it is best to take a vow of silence. Otherwise, if you talk negatively to others, you will collect more karma instead of burning it. Be in complete silence. Silence is not to speak nor to write. If you are writing, that is not total silence. Avoid even writing or being on the phone or texting unless it is to communicate an emergency. Emergencies are exceptions. But when I see people doing silence, I see them writing and communicating with others most of the time. They are not speaking, but they are writing, so it is the same thing. What are words? Communication. And what is writing? Communication. I suggest that if anger and negativities attack you, to be in complete silence. The anger will subdue, and you will not collect more karma.

Remember that fasting is not a competition. People who compete in fasting just create more ego and problems for themselves. It is wrong. I have seen it with Jain monks and nuns in India. They say, "He did 100 days, so I'm going to do it too." So, they try to do it, and sadly, sometimes they die. Sometimes it takes only eight days to die when forcing a fast because their body was maybe only able to do four days. Don't try to compete with others. Don't compare yourself. Go according to your own body, and you will benefit more. When people become too extreme, others get turned off by this valuable and ancient spiritual practice.

When you fast to compete or for physical reasons, you will be missing out on the most significant benefit. I am not opposed to fasting for physical reasons. But you will only experience a small benefit. Remember what I told you at the beginning of the book: the real word for fasting is upavaasa, which means to reside close to your soul. It means you focus on your soul with the sole purpose of awakening yourself, becoming purer, and becoming totally karma-less. Your soul's real nature is right knowledge, right vision, and right conduct. The soul is already in bliss, and you need to connect with it. In upavaasa, you drop your lower qualities, bad habits, bad behavior, worldly taste, worldly things, and worldly anything.

The biggest benefit of upavaasa is the purification of your body, mind, and soul. This is the real transformation. The real healing. And the real liberation. You experience having a light body, and a light body allows you to enter a full meditative state - the state your soul deeply craves. The soul is waiting for you. You can experience this extraordinary phenomenon. Once you get there, you experience your soul. The soul needs to burn all the karma, and when karma is burned, nothing can make you suffer. If you have not yet experienced your soul, have patience. It means there is karma on the way, and it might require more time to burn it.

You have to go little by little, but your destiny gets straighten out when you burn your karma. Your death and birth cycle end. If karma continues to surround your soul, no matter how good you are, it will create blockages and suffering in your life. Follow my advice and recommendations so you can fast the right way. If you do it the right way, you will not have trouble, and you will achieve your goal – to liberate your soul. The removal of karma sets your soul free, and you are almost there.

ABOUT THE AUTHOR

Acharya Shree Yogeesh is a living enlightened master of this era and is the founder of the Siddhayatan Tirth and Spiritual Retreat, a unique 250+ acre spiritual pilgrimage site and meditation park in North America providing the perfect atmosphere for spiritual learning, community, and soul awakening to help truth seekers advance spiritually. Acharya Shree is also the founder of the Yogeesh Ashram International in India, Yogeesh Ashram near Los Angeles, California, Siddhayatan Mandir Estonia in Europe, and the Acharya Yogeesh Primary & Higher Secondary children's school in Haryana, India.

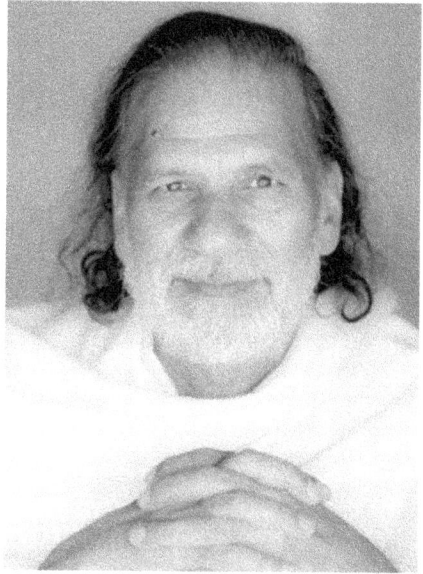

As an inspiring revolutionary spiritual leader and in-demand speaker worldwide, for nearly fifty years Acharya Shree has dedicated his life to helping guide hundreds of thousands of people on their spiritual journeys of self-improvement and self-realization.

It is Acharya Shree's mission to spread the message of nonviolence, vegetarianism, oneness, and total transformation.

Meet him at Siddhayatan.org and connect with him via social media on Instagram, Facebook and YouTube: @AcharyaShreeYogeesh.

- Also by Acharya Shree Yogeesh -

Awaken!
A Handbook for the Truth Seeker

Secrets of Enlightenment
Volume I

Secrets of Enlightenment
Volume II

Chakra Awakening:
The Lost Techniques

Soulful Wisdom & Art
101 Though-Provoking Quotes
for Inspiration and Transformation

Soul Talks
New Beginnings

Soul Talks
The Path of Purification

Soul Talks
The Power of Intention

ACKNOWLEDGMENTS

The words "Thank You" are not enough to extend to Sadhvi Anubhuti for the hard and special work she did to make this book come to life. She tirelessly put her heart and soul into making this book the best it can be. Not only did she transcribe and compile my talks giving her a lot of confidence, she has also understood the deeper teachings behind fasting that will help her to guide others in this practice. Expect more writing from her in the future.

I cannot say "Thank You" enough to Sadhvi Siddhali Shree who continues to publish books to help spread the teachings. Without her, this book and all my other work, would not have taken any shape at all and reach your eyes and hands.

My third "Thank You" goes to our pillar of Siddhayatan Tirth, Riddhika Nadler -- she has done a fantastic job by reading the proof and making corrections.

I hope this book will make a big impact on its readers.

CONNECT WITH US

Siddhayatan Spiritual Retreat Center

with Water Fasting Retreats

https://siddhayatan.org

YouTube

https://youtube.com/acharyashreeyogeesh

Instagram

https://instagram.com/acharyashreeyogeesh

The ACHARYA SHREE YOGEESH Podcast

iTunes - Spotify - Pandora

Fasting + Guidance

https://thefastingbook.com

https://instagram.com/thefastingbook

INDEX

INDEX

INDEX

INDEX

INDEX

INDEX

INDEX

INDEX

INDEX